THE
INTERPRETATION
OF ILLNESS

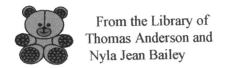
THE
INTERPRETATION
OF ILLNESS

by
Frederic D. Homer

Purdue University Press
West Lafayette, Indiana

Library of Congress Cataloging-in-Publication Data

Homer, Frederic D.
  The interpretation of illness

  1. Medicine, Psychosomatic. 2. Psychoanalytic
interpretation. 3. Self-disclosure. 4. Groddeck, Georg,
1866–1934. I. Title. [DNLM: 1. Groddeck, Georg,
1866–1934. 2. Attitude to Health—correspondence.
2. Psychoanalysis—correspondence. 3. Psychoanalytic
Interpretation—correspondence. WM 460.7 H766i]
RC49.H63   1987   616.89   87–7221
ISBN 0–911198–88–1 (pbk.)

Published in 1988
Printed in the United States of America
Book and cover designed by Lynn Gastinger

Table of Contents

Preface

Illness is a communication to others. None of us consciously likes to be sick or hurt, but we all, consciously or unconsciously, tell others about our ills. Others then extend sympathy. If we change this pattern of communication by learning to forgo sympathy or to gain it in less destructive ways, we can prevent illness or alleviate existing symptoms. These ideas were inspired by philosopher-physician Georg Groddeck who insisted that we cause and hence can cure organic illness in ourselves. This work takes Groddeck's initial insight about illness and makes it a starting point for self-inquiry comparable to Sigmund Freud's analysis of dreams. Freud gave us an understanding of the dream as well as its relation to the psyche. This essay will give an understanding of illness as well as an alternative to Freud's view of inner life.

Georg Groddeck corresponded with his contemporary Freud and was one of the few to whom Freud acknowledged a debt. In *The Ego and the Id,* Freud thanks Groddeck for introducing him to the idea of the *it* from which Freud derived the *id.* Groddeck was known and respected as a great healer in spite of a strained relationship with psychoanalysts and psychoanalytic societies of his day. Due to this estrangement, few of his contemporaries, with the exception of Freud and a small following, acknowledged his ideas.

Today, empirical research by Hans Selye and his followers links psychological stress and illness, the relationship Groddeck anticipated in the nineteen twenties. Stress theory, although extremely useful, lacks the specificity of Groddeck's theory into the psychodynamics of illness. Groddeck could understand what individual differences might cause one person and not another to be ill in similar stressful circumstances. His concept of the unconscious (the it) provides for the possibility of a more extensive self-inquiry into the psyche and illness than do many other theories. In addition, Groddeck's research shows why contemporary practices—from faith healing to biofeedback to stress counseling—cure, but only on a hit-or-miss basis.

The Interpretation of Illness develops a climate of sympathy and understanding for Groddeck's thought; I gather and sort through his ideas on the structure of the psyche, the nature of illness, and the methods of self-analysis. A key difference between my thought and Groddeck's surfaces: I cannot proceed as Groddeck does by devaluating *awareness.* For Groddeck, the it is the ruling force of the psyche; the feeling one has of being *I* is merely a trick of the *it.* In contrast, for me, conscious awareness is the door to inner life. Perhaps our disagreement is a matter of philosophical temperament, often the cornerstone of all philosophical differences. I can admire, but not emulate, the studied passivity of Groddeck towards *life.*

After my disquisition on Groddeck, I undertake self-inquiry, and my starting point is free association used in conjunction with Groddeck's favorite question: what are the consequences of your illness? I develop other methods of access to the psyche along with concepts that describe inner life: the *self, life, awareness, difference, blessings, curses, reveries, ruminations, sympathy,* and *annihilation.* What I unveil is the elegant simplicity of the psychoanalytic method and the utter complexity of its data. When the promise of psychoanalysis—knowledge is cure—does not alleviate symptoms, I introduce into self-inquiry the techniques of family therapists.

I conclude that an understanding of the language and of the dynamics of illness is the cornerstone for the broader task of learning to express ourselves to others with *clarity* and *candor.* Not only do physical symptoms abate but also we feel a full rush of freedom. Freedom does not come to the existentialist suffering alone, but it comes to those of us who express ourselves deliberately and knowingly to others.

Once again, with respect to the style of this book, I begin with an idea of Groddeck's only to develop my own. Groddeck wrote his major work, *The Book of the It,* as a series of letters from Patrik Troll to a friend. The letters enabled Groddeck to be as structured in his thoughts as he needed to be and at the same time provided him a vehicle for his free associations and analyses. I too adopt the letter form, and using the persona August "Augie" Sayres, I write letters to several people because that technique allows me to practice the idea of speaking directly to others with candor. By speaking simultaneously to the I and the it of another person, I can express myself with the linear precision of the analytic philosopher and through the metaphor of the poet. The letter, a form borrowed from the humanities, enhances the existential practice of personalized yet rigorously philosophical vision. A postcursor to existential tradition, *The Interpretation of Illness* uses Augie's adventures to personalize theory and method, emphasizing the phenomenological aspects of life and awareness that speak to the concerns of others. In two instances, I do use the essay form to express my thoughts. One essay introduces the reader to Groddeck's thoughts, and a bit further in the text, an address to the graduating class of a medical school tells doctors how the ideas expressed in this work may invigorate traditional medical practice.

Although my task is structurally similar to Freud's and the initial insight is Groddeck's, this work will be grounded in my own social and intellectual context. In my earlier work *Guns and Garlic: Myths and Realities of Organized Crime,* I study flawed characters. My interests progressed to an examination of *character* in an analytical and historical way. In my book *Character,* I study the manifold possibilities of human existence: a perspective that encourages us to look unblinkingly at our limits. Philosophy and heroism are indistinguishable for me. *The Interpretation of Illness* also pushes to the limits of possibility. The boundary condition of death that frames and limits our existence is more within our responsibility and control than we were heretofore aware. Through this study, I will show that minute by minute, often below the level of awareness, we are making choices about life and death, health and illness. The ruling passion in this work, as in my others, is an existential one: we must become overseers and not victims of our own existence. This is the philosophical nest on which this study rests.

The two poles of *sympathy* and *annihilation* are the context for my metapsychology. We are seeking either of these aims constantly. I argue that except for brief moments neither one is attainable. We are incomplete beings, and through increasing awareness, we must reconcile ourselves to our tenuousness with others and the world. We must choose to understand our difference in a world which is much as the philosopher Georg Simmel describes: a conflict, a struggle, a series of difficult choices.

In my previous work *Character,* the development of *character* starts with *integrity:* the identification with the critical ideas of others while not giving up on our own thoughts as the center. Ideas of *importance* to us, built on *reverie* and *reflection,* begin to intrude to establish our *difference* with others. Finally, we *return* to the world on our own terms. This process describes the rhythm of this work.

The Interpretation of Illness begins with an exploration of Groddeck's ideas, experiments with my own methods and concepts, and then becomes deliberate again as I return with my own thoughts about illness as a communication. The book is about ideas and their exploration. Use the book as a springboard for free association; let your it as well as your I react. Read slowly in a relaxed mood, find new avenues of access to the psyche, and return to the world with a new synthesis.

For those more visually inclined, to read the letters and essays without a description of the author would be unsatisfactory. Augie is forty-six years old, lives in Wyoming, and is a professor at the university in Laramie. He is six feet two inches tall, has green eyes, and a calm facade that masks inner intensity. Augie is well aware of the paradox of appearing a bit warmer and more personable to those who know him than he does in letters that explore how people might communicate directly with each other.

Those most influential in the formulation of this work are Lawrence Durrell, Nikos Kazantzakis, Ortega y Gasset, Henri Bergson, William James, Georg Simmel, Gabriel Marcel, Elias Canetti, Gregory Bateson, Rollo May, Jay Haley, Cloe Madanes, Sal Minuchin, Stephen Jay Gould, Michel Foucault, and Carl Rogers.

Letter to B. J.

AuGUST SAYRES
MEDICINE Bow, WYOMING

Dear B. J.,

I must tell you of my recent acquaintance with the work of an extraordinary man, Georg Walther Groddeck. At present I am racing ahead to find out all I can about his life and ideas. As a tease, let me suggest that one of his fundamental ideas is that we cause all of our own illnesses and injuries. This idea is embedded in a comprehensive set of ideas about life and existence. Groddeck was a contemporary of Freud and was known for his power to cure organic illnesses.

I said "a tease" because for complete information you will have to await my biography of Groddeck. To get you started, however, I enclose my Introduction to the biography. Unfortunately for my research, his works are difficult to find in America. In England, where I am at present, you can find his works if you look hard. A friend of mine brought Groddeck's name to my attention several years ago. Mike is very clever and knew that I would eventually search out Groddeck and make him my own. Let me tell you about my ideas in recent years and how Groddeck now fits in.

I recently published a book called *Character.* In it I survey flawed characters in America in order to suggest a model of character which would serve as a vehicle for living well. The concept of character, in turn, helps to evaluate our social system. This exploration delineated the basic agony of philosophy for me. As my study of character helped me to achieve my freedom from social and political restraints, so did this inquiry acutely point out the limits of my freedom: a freedom circumscribed by actions of the conventional and the bizarre characters that surround us.

The details of the work are unimportant here, but *Character* led me to explore the social system and allowed me to make my uneasy truce with it. In the final chapters of that book, I began to use the word *candor* to describe a stance that one should

3

achieve towards the world. We should come to the world on our own terms, with candor, whenever possible. There should be a consonance between the way we think and we live. We should not live with secret consciousness, a set of ideas we keep to ourselves, while projecting false personas on the world.

As I finished the book, I saw that the concepts of character and candor presupposed the existence of the answers to a prior question: are we candid with ourselves? This made me ripe for psychoanalytic thought again, and I took up anew with Freud and successively C. G. Jung, Melanie Klein, Rollo May, Karen Horney, Carl Rogers, R. D. Laing, and Thomas Szasz, as well as others. With my emphasis on an exploration of candor, I was ready for the works of yet another psychoanalyst, one like Groddeck who was also philosopher and physician.

The philosopher Groddeck intrigued me because, as you know, I am modestly engaged in the enterprise of erecting my own philosophical edifice. *Character* is one outcome of such studies. Groddeck's philosophy was immediately appealing for he was a philosopher who concentrated on my next question, candor. As you know, B. J., I presently teach the sociology of mental illness. Consequently, the physician Groddeck's proposition that we cause our own illnesses and injuries was attractive to me because I have studied the long history of illness and its various causes.

I know all that sounds too summary and "objective" to be the way all my thoughts folded into place. It sounds like a rationalization for why I am writing *Georg Groddeck: A Biography* now. Nonetheless, the foregoing are the reasons why *Groddeck* is important to me and ultimately will work as a book.

Now, if I may give you the history of the idea, it might seem more authentic. I was browsing in the small library at Maria Assumpta in Kensington, where I am presently teaching a group of American students. I spotted Groddeck's *Book of the It* on the shelves. In truth, I had earlier looked at psychoanalytic literature in bookstores and libraries, hoping to spot Groddeck. I flipped through the pages and quickly lost track of time and place. Here it was: we create our own organic illnesses. I had, in some recesses of my mind, known this all along. Now I had a friend, a colleague. Not only a psychologist, but a philosopher, a literary critic, and a person, in my terms, who had character. Groddeck was a person with integrity and a sense of what was important, and he returned to the world on his own terms.

Since then, I have been absorbed in little else. I have delved into the related areas of biology, medicine, and everything from the supernatural to the viral that pretends to cause and suggests cure of illness. My studies were also prompted by serious illness (coronary bypass surgery), as well as the usual string of minor to major ailments that we all seem to suffer with stoic resignation, the "victims of external forces." With my existential leanings, the thought of controlling my own illnesses had manifold possibilities. What a wonderful juncture at which to expand my own freedom, to push back the boundaries of death and disease that threaten my life. Like similar struggles, this one is not without seeing limits to existence, but that is another story. The heroic is to extend the limits of freedom while keeping vigilant to other limits that freedom makes manifest.

The reading of Groddeck suggested a response to illness quite different from the one I write about in *Will and Recovery*. In that work, with which I am still pleased, I conclude that knowing our own life and circumstances will allow for command over our own illness and recovery. In the book, I show how we can gain control over the unfamiliar (doctors, hospitals, social isolation, and technology) to make critical choices. I never realized at that time how far over the domain of illness our influence could reach. *Groddeck* will extend my analysis and greatly enhance it.

Groddeck did not want disciples. My biography of him is addressed more to possibilities in his writing than to a canonization of the man and his ideas. He understood my idea that character is not imitation. As I write the pages in *Groddeck,* I see all kinds of possibilities. I will be corresponding to you about some of them. My sister says that I am very suggestible. Yesterday I was James and even Emerson; today I am Groddeck. I do live and enjoy their ideas, and then the inevitable difference sets in. I am all I read and see, I am none—of my own choosing. What will follow after *Groddeck* is my own philosophy.

Now you know why I have been so silent. First, I was ill; and as is customary in my family, we eschew sympathy, pretend to bravery, keep illness to ourselves. After convalescence and writing *Will and Recovery,* I have been submerged in Groddeck and his friends.

Augie Sayres

PS. Perhaps my current interests can be explained by an expression my grandmother often used: ''Your health comes first—you can always hang yourself later.''

Georg Groddeck:
A Biography

by
August Sayres

Introduction

There is a good deal of difficulty in writing a biography about Georg Walther Groddeck (1866–1934) because he warns a would-be biographer away from the task. In his most comprehensive book, *The Book of the It,* he suggests that if we like what he says we should look at life anew through our own lenses. The only way to write a biography of Groddeck in accordance with his wishes is to emphasize a world open to possibility. In this biography, I attempt to organize Groddeck's ideas in the way they helped me to look anew at the world. What I can best hope to achieve in this work is to convince the reader to study Groddeck in his or her own way. The philosopher, physician, psychologist, poet, art critic, and literary critic will each see him in a different fashion, for he practiced all these skills and contributed to an understanding of each.

Groddeck was trained as a physician and wrote of experiences in his practice. He felt obligations to individuals, but not to schools of thought. He was well read in many areas and made many contributions to his field, but he was often neglected because he ignored or criticized the methodological canons and restrictive jargon used in the research of his time. He was criticized for not being scientific at a time when those who were developing psychoanalysis were staking claims to its scientific status.

If Groddeck is known at all, it is for two reasons. First, he applied with great success the principles of psychoanalysis to organic illness. Second, underlying his treatment was his idea of the *it,* a congerie of unknown and mostly unknowable forces within the person that affect everything from breathing, digestion, and the development of organic diseases to outward manifestations of behavior—even the *I,* or consciousness. What I intend to do in this introduction is to place these and other aspects of his broad perspective within a framework that is useful

9

to my own thought. The ensuing chapters elaborate on his ideas and will manifest my own disagreements with and departures from them.

Please remember that this biography is no substitute for reading Groddeck's own work, which is far less an attempt at a system than this study. His work expresses his thought through poetry of language, metaphor, and diverse associations. Those who write about him are tied to the illusion (his term) that the I, or ego, is governor of thoughts and actions. His writings, especially *The Book of the It,* make few attempts to mask the fundamental processes of the it. Grasping this difference between Groddeck and others is fundamental for an appreciation of his thoughts. Most readers are turned off by his use of metaphor, his unwillingness to systematize, his long rambling sections of associations, and his unwillingness to conform to the canons of social science. If we read him with the understanding that his method is not carelessness but an exposition on how the it works, then we can fully appreciate his work. When reading Groddeck, we must pretend that he drew up the rules of exposition and all attempts at systematization are pretences of the I to sovereignty over the it.

First, I will look at his ideas about the *integrity* of persons, their basic structure and being. Here I will explore what he meant by the it and the I. Second, I will investigate how the meager I can find out what is *important* about its own life and circumstances so as to know how to act. Finally, I will show how the individual is supposed to *return* to the world of others and act towards them. These categories are not analytically distinct but overlap each other.

Groddeck was born and lived in Germany. He spent most of his adult life in the town of Baden-Baden where he practised medicine that became heavily directed towards treating terminally ill patients. Although he was German, his patriotic identifications were not strong. At one time, he commented that there were Germans, Frenchmen, and Groddecks. He always felt different and had no need for group identification.

His father was a physician, and a chance remark about what a good observation young Georg made, "just like a physician," influenced him to choose a career in medicine. Groddeck trained under Bismarck's physician, Ernst Schweninger, and patterned his techniques after those of his mentor: diet, massage, hot baths, and authoritative commands. On his own, Groddeck developed techniques of analysis that helped him to understand the unconscious (it) forces in a person that cause the person to become ill. Some time later, he discovered Sigmund Freud's writings, which covered some of the same ground. After the initial disappointment of finding himself not unique in his discoveries, he enthusiastically took on many of Freud's methods and, mainly through correspondence, developed a constructive relationship with Freud. Many of Groddeck's works were published through the auspices of the psychoanalytic society with the approval of Freud and Otto Rank. He gained a wide reputation as a healer, and Freud acknowledged in *The Ego and the Id* that Groddeck was influential in the development of the ideas in that book.

Groddeck's reputation as a successful healer spread through the psychoanalytic community, but it was hampered by his relationships with individual members. Groddeck refused to adhere to the canons of science and regarded the use of jargon with contempt. At one of the few psychoanalytic conventions he attended, he announced that he was the "wild analyst" and proceeded to free associate (it-talk) throughout his presentation.

We are the better for his estrangement from the movement. He developed and maintained his ideas independently. Groddeck acknowledged a large debt to the writings of Freud but refused to modify his own views. In his correspondence, Groddeck shows regret at Freud's misunderstanding and modification of his concept of the it (which became Freud's concept of the id). Much of the discussion in Groddeck's letters is aimed at winning Freud's full approval of his views, something that was not forthcoming. Freud, on the other hand, tried to draw Groddeck into the orthodox fold. As they grew older, Groddeck pleaded with Freud to visit him in Baden-Baden. Although Groddeck never said so directly, he felt he could cure Freud's cancer of the jaw. This would have been the ultimate justification of Groddeck's work. Freud never made the trip.

This brief overview places Groddeck, who was also influenced by the vitalists and Nietzsche, in a historical perspective. Like most biographers feel about their subject, I feel that Groddeck and his works have been greatly overlooked. It may be helpful to examine his ambivalent status in the psychoanalytic community, the audience that could make or break his reputation. The members of that community certainly could not accept him as a cofounder with Freud; he refused to alter his own beliefs and cooperate in the "larger goals" of the psychoanalytic movement. Furthermore, he was firm in his own methods that leaned more heavily on a vitalist position laced with skepticism than on the use of scientific methods. Finally, Freud was interested in an elaboration of neuroses and staked out a narrow, specialized claim to the treatment of disease. Freud's acceptance of Groddeck's idea might have undermined the credibility of his own carefully orchestrated campaign to make psychoanalysis respectable. Further, making the it the basis of all illness would have relativized Freud's thought and made his substantive concerns with neurosis a narrow subfield in the vast terrain of Groddeck.

We cannot blame Freud for Groddeck's obscurity. Freud published Groddeck's works, encouraged him to join in his activities, and gave him a forum. Groddeck made the choice to go his own way, and although "he protests too much," Groddeck appeared to thrive on and even be pleased by his independence.

Groddeck worked inductively, developing his ideas from his practice. These ideas are primarily contained in four books: *The Book of the It, The Unknown Self, Exploring the Unconscious,* and *The World of Man.* Written in the form of letters to a friend, the first work is the most comprehensive rendering of his ideas. He explores ideas from his own cases or his own experiences and is almost apologetic if he runs on too long about a formal concept. The second and third books are collections of papers, articles printed for his patients; and the fourth work is made up of fragments that were to have been part of a longer work.

Like William James and Ralph Waldo Emerson before him, Groddeck was interested in capturing the richness and variety of existence. He also retained the privilege of changing his mind. Consequently, expressing Groddeck's ideas in a systematic manner is a tricky business. As Groddeck might have predicted, a synthesis may be more my thoughts than his. The reduction of discussions of the it and other concepts to an analytic language without his rich use of metaphor both gains and loses. On the one hand, such a treatment forms the basis for comparison with other philosophers; on the other, it restricts his ideas.

To assume that Groddeck was sloppy, careless, or solely inductive is misleading. Many of his critics found him unscientific and even mystical. As with Emerson and James, his method was not to confuse and obfuscate existence but to take care not to oversimplify reality for the sake of a system. His suggestion that much is unknown or unknowable should not be taken as mysticism but as the attitude of someone careful about generalizing from evidence and modest in his claims about existence, someone who has a healthy scientific skepticism. What Groddeck lacked, and this threw him out of step with his contemporaries, was enlightened optimism about science and man, what Abraham Kaplan calls the ordinal fallacy. If today we know X about the world through science, tomorrow we will know Y and Z as well, for science is young and its methods are yet to be perfected. Groddeck did not share that optimism, nor did he feel that knowledge was a straight road to mastery or virtue.

Integrity

Henri Bergson suggests that at the core of every philosophy is a simple idea and all the rest is commentary on that idea. In Groddeck's writings, there is always a recurrence of the idea of the it. He viewed the it as central to his thought and the basis for treatment of his patients. He was greatly disappointed when Freud used this concept in *The Ego and the Id* and changed its meaning. Like the other vitalists, Groddeck chose to view life from within. What he sensed was a vast array of forces, or life, if you will, that moved the individual. These forces predate the development of the I-feeling, or consciousness, in the individual. The it is present when the sperm and egg join, cells begin to multiply, and organs begin to form. Even as adults, much of life is conducted below consciousness. The body manufactures red blood cells, breaks down foods, injures itself, takes ill, creates itches, makes gestures, performs a whole range of activity. The it, for Groddeck, was much more inclusive than the unconscious, which was described by others as what was known and is now forgotten or, in psychoanalytic language, repressed. The it is life, and much of the it is unknown to us and is likely to remain unknowable.

People have assumed that Groddeck was a mystic. He was no more a mystic than those before him who followed the Delphic injunction to know thyself and came up wanting. In his thinking, Groddeck appears to have followed Bergson's lead on these issues. Generally, Groddeck argues that we can only know life through our intuition and that many of these life processes will remain unknown or unknowable to us. This was a revolt against the mechanistic science of Herbert Spencer and Charles Darwin, who concluded that we live in a world where behavior is determined by outside forces and where science gives a series of static pictures of change depicted in space. Despite his protestations, Groddeck does not reject mechanistic science altogether. Science is where he must get his evidence about conception, the function of internal organs, and circulation of the blood. Perhaps he might best be described as a skeptical vitalist. To learn about the it is to know about life, but direct access to the it is limited.

Near the end of *The Book of the It,* Groddeck further complicates his idea. Early in the book, he ascribes the word *es,* or *it,* to this phenomenon because the word is as amorphous as the concept. He does not want the it to be encompassed by a one-line definition or a simple metaphor. He tries to capture phases of the it with a continuous stream of metaphors. At times, the it is a troll, trying to trick consciousness; at other times, the it is not mischievous but benevolent, trying to help out consciousness by making the organism ill and taking the I from a threatening situation; still at other times, the it is merely a blind mechanical association responding deterministically to stimuli. Groddeck has many more images of the it. All of them seem to reflect the poet's wish to see all facets of the subject rather than to settle for one definition. At this juncture, the scientist might jump in and ask: without a model how can we predict human behavior? Groddeck's answer is that we cannot understand cause and to do so would be to give a distorted picture of the it. We cannot precisely predict how the it works. All we can do is poke and prod around hoping to bring changes in behavior. Groddeck leaves the it to its mysterious ways.

This does not mean that Groddeck's metaphors and his explanations of why we get sick are without utility. With each explanation, he tries to determine the consequences that derive from the it's behavior. When he says, for instance, that the it returns us to the infant's position of power, or exacts pity from others, he is suggesting how the it might work. To the scientist, he is perhaps able to explain everything and hence explain nothing. One must ask if Groddeck's tolerance for ambiguity might not be as useful in scientific investigation as the stance of those who posit instincts, needs, or motives with certainty, only to be contradicted by others or to change their own mind and move from certainty to certainty. Groddeck was not locked into Jean-Jacques Rousseau's natural sympathy; Thomas Hobbes's power; Freud's eros, thanatos, pleasure principle, reality principle; or any of the manifold instincts, drives, and sentiments hitherto or hence posited. Much of Groddeck's work is fixed not on determining cause, but on the pragmatist's question: what are the consequences of the impulses of the it?

In the last letters of *The Book of the It,* Groddeck further complicates his description of the it. We were under the impression that the it is being for Groddeck, a monolith that is existence for him. If society is God for Emile Durkheim, the it is sovereign for Groddeck. We find out later, however, that the it is not an it, but its. Groddeck moves to polytheism. There may be a belly it and a liver it; each cell may even have an it, as with the co-joined sperm and egg at conception. Groddeck anticipates here what others have found with respect to genetic structures.

As with the choice to describe the it in a variegated metaphorical way, the decision to have a polytheistic it has interesting consequences. Groddeck avoids the mind-body dichotomy because there is no central locus for the governor, or ego. Power is decentralized and different coalitions of its may act or rule at different times. He anticipates the difficulties that doctors and scientists have when they try to define the cessation of life. For most of them, brain death is not sufficient. Groddeck would agree that many other its are still active even when the brain is dead.

Most important for his medical practice, Groddeck's refusal to dichotomize mind and body and his positing of an infinity of its allow him to avoid the split between psychological and organic disease. We are now used to this dichotomy. We assume that psychologists, through a talking cure of one sort or another, can get rid of "psychological problems," or problems arising from internal causes. One of these psychological problems may be psychosomatic diseases. We also assume that doctors, using methodist techniques practiced since the early Roman empire, can administer medicines to alleviate "organic problems," or problems stemming from external causes such as viruses and bacteria.

We tend to forget that throughout most of medical history no distinction has been made between mind and body. Holistic medicine today is merely the rediscovery of an approach known through the ages. The sharp distinction came at the end of the classical period when certain diseases were viewed as moral defects. Because of the influence of Philippe Pinel and especially William Tuke, the soul was treated through discipline and punishment. Freud and the psychoanalysts maintained this distinction and divided the practice of caring for people into mind and body. Freud, trained as a physician, eventually began to treat hysteria. He became a practitioner of the mind and allowed lay analysts like Theodor Reik and Rank to practice.

Groddeck's conception of the it followed those who made no distinction between mind and body. His idea of illness was more like that of Schweninger, his mentor, than that of Freud. This is illustrated by Schweninger's method of treatment by diet, baths, and authoritative commands. Correspondingly, Groddeck did not label a disease as either of the mind or of the body. A patient might be treated for a red throat, fever, convulsions, and disorientation. For Schweninger and Groddeck, these symptoms were not viewed as body distinct from mind.

Groddeck used the language of organic illness and psychological illness mostly because he was speaking to the practitioners who used that language. Only with orthodox psychoanalysts did he bother to distinguish organic from psychological illness to differentiate his contribution from theirs. He preferred to make no distinction at all; and to use our modern terminology, if he cured a patient's sore throat through a talking cure, he also cured a problem that the patient had in living and understanding himself. Also, remember that he retained the therapy of diet and massage in treatment.

His understanding that there were a multiplicity of its also kept him from a labeling perspective on disease. Its could combine in infinite ways to incapacitate the whole organism. There were belly diseases and other combinations of diseased its that ignored traditional diagnoses. He occasionally used labels but never lost sight of the multiplicity of symptoms (in today's dichotomous language) both mental and physical that are associated with one another. A coughing sound might be in tandem with the reception of an unpleasant remark, cramps, or a desire to flee a social situation. A headache and the appearance of an old adversary might coincide with extreme fidgeting and heavy perspiration.

With an understanding of the it, we are now prepared to treat the core of Groddeck's philosophy. Groddeck suggests that we are lived by the it. This life force, the it, starts at conception (perhaps further back), constructs our spleen, liver, heart, and even our brain. Most significant: the it creates the I. In most theories, the I (or ego or consciousness) is the governing force, sometimes in opposition to unconscious forces but in command or aspiring to command. Groddeck gives much more primacy to the it (or the unconscious forces) and proposes that the I is the tool of the it, a trick of the it, and certainly the child of the it. Although we have different images of the I in Groddeck, the I is consistently subordinate to the it. He suggests that the feeling that I am I—this verdict we all come to—is necessary. We are compelled to believe this, so we can believe we control our own life and the lives of others. For Groddeck, this is merely an illusion, because we are lived by the it.

In *The Book of the It,* he goes further to posit that the I wishes to believe that the organism has no parents and no connections to others in the universe. Not only does the I proclaim its sovereignty over the organism, but also wants to take credit for the origins of the organism. This latter argument seems to be an implicit criticism of Nietzsche's *Zarathustra*. When Groddeck indicates that we are lived through the it, he is saying that the it lets the I think it is sovereign.

Groddeck's views about the relationship of the it to the I have profound implications for the rest of his theory. First, his vitalism depends on the I getting to know the it, or life. The problem is that our knowledge of the it is dependent on the I, yet the I is not an autonomous governor of the organism. When I call Groddeck a skeptical vitalist, it is for this reason.

Epistemologically, we know through our understanding of the it as gathered by the I. However, the I as a tool of the it is not a trustworthy reporter of the truth. We can see now where Groddeck's skepticism about science comes from. A community of judges deciding on what truth is may be a community of I's all being tricked in the same way.

Groddeck does not give a systematic solution to this problem of epistemology, but his thought suggests answers. One way of dealing with this is through an ironic stance in which we are almost mocking our findings in the next paragraph. Another way to grapple with the problem of being lived by the it is to try to discover how the it made the organism ill. Groddeck felt that although the organism is always ill in some way, through access to the it he might come to cure many of these ills.

Finally, Groddeck attempts to communicate directly with himself and others in the language of the it. He firmly believed that when we talk to one another, our its are doing the communicating. We could also get in touch with our own it by going directly to the language of association and metaphor. In this sense, life and truth were both the it. He was fond of saying that the it never lied. The it made associations and did not differentiate between object and symbol; this was not a lie to him. A penis might be a sausage which might be a tall building which might also be a woman's finger. We might get at truth and being if we drop much of the pretense of the I and learn the rules of the it. All associations are true for the it.

Beware, this is a systematic reconstruction of many fragments in Groddeck, but perhaps this inquiry can be productive.

Let me begin with a digression on the prior sentence, because the sentence provides me with an example of how Groddeck feels we communicate in it-talk and not through what the I intentionally expresses. In the sentence where I suggest that I will tie Groddeck's fragments together, I am describing a rational procedure. In that sentence, my it is saying, "I am doing a difficult job. I am contributing something original in the analysis. I am smarter than Groddeck." This is quite different from what my I thought was the purpose of the sentence.

Groddeck says that one person's it communicates with the it of another. Without my tutelage, you might have ignored the sentence, taken the sentence to mean the same as it meant to my it, associated the archaeological metaphor "systematic reconstruction of many fragments" with futile attempts as a child to learn from fragments of the past about the present, sympathized with Groddeck because the phrase "fragments in Groddeck" reminds you of a pane of glass you broke that wounded you with fragments—or your it could drum up any of thousands of possibilities.

This method of it-talk, rich in association and metaphor, reminds me of the way that Milton Erickson would deliberately communicate with his patients. For Erickson, this method was a way through reason to place suggestions to the patient below the level of consciousness. His hypnotic suggestions were Groddeck's it-talk. So much of Groddeck's work, especially his *Book of the It* and *World of Man,* is an attempt to speak through the language of the it. Groddeck felt that messages would be variously received, depending on the associations of the other's it. Also, for Groddeck, it-talk meant that much of the suggestion one person makes to another is not a matter of conscious calculation, rather one it composes to another it. My it composed that sentence "Beware, this is a systematic reconstruction . . ." for your it.

For Groddeck, in this sense, the it might be a troll. The it creates the I and feeds it purposeful statements, all of which obscure the true communication of the organism. The I is a dupe of the it, as is the I of the person being spoken to. If I say, "It's been nice talking to you, but I have to go to the store now," my it may be saying, "The store is a great refuge from you (as it was from my parents). It was very uncomfortable talking to you." In this sense, for Groddeck, the it, as always, speaks the truth; however, the I is deluded and lies.

An ideal situation would be to understand how the it works and then to get the I to be aware of how the I is the tool of the it. The I could be put more directly in the service of the it. You may say to a friend, "Take this job. It is a piece of cake." He may hate cake because of a traumatic birthday when his mother forgot to get him a cake, and he has since denied that he was upset about not getting one. Your it may have heard his it saying that he did not want the job and remembered his saying he hated cake. Even though the I-message is to take the job, the it-message is to turn down the job. If we are consciously aware of these processes, we can more effectively communicate with our own self and others.

It-talk does not fully extricate Groddeck from his difficulties. We still have the possibility that the I, in trying to understand the it, is being deceived by the it. It-talk and understanding it-language, if we could believe the I in this instance, could help us to understand life and truth. But, communication with others still remains difficult. Even if the I can be used more in the service of the it to understand another's it and to compose in language deliberately made to be understood by the other person's it, communication is still poor. The richness of association of the other's it does not permit the assurance that we will be understood in the way we want. Groddeck is very much aware of this problem. A story he tells of a patient illustrates this very well. A patient continually came to him with complaints of physical ailments. He said to her that she probably got sick only because she wanted to see a doctor. His I meant this remark as a rueful joke. She did not return to him for treatment. Twenty years later she called to tell him he was right. Since that time, she had never been ill or gone to a doctor. Groddeck, of course, had forgotten the incident. Here was a happy coincidence of it speaking to it with Groddeck's I unaware. Just as likely, another patient could have taken that statement as a sign that Groddeck did not like him or her and gone to another doctor with even more frequency, or tried any one of a number of solutions.

In sum, Groddeck offers three ways to deal with the problem that we are lived through the it: irony, the futile quest for the I to know the it, or the granting of free expression to the it. We never completely get around the problem of truth residing with the it and not the I, yet we always proceed as if the I is sovereign. Even an ironic stance presupposes that the I knows with certainty that the I is controlled by the it.

The centrality of the it and the awareness of the I are focal concepts for Groddeck. Given this framework, we may ask how we know about the external world. In the very first essay he writes in his *Book of the It,* he admits to sharing his father's skepticism of knowledge. Science, for Groddeck, would be knowledge the I shares with the other I's that are looking at the same problem. This knowledge is not trustworthy. Discipline might train a person to be more aware of the it, hence of the I, and consequently be a better scientist than someone else. But Groddeck makes no effort at all to justify science on these grounds.

He does, however, rely on verifiable scientific knowledge to describe conception and the function of the liver and other organs. Groddeck never denies that we can have knowledge of the "outside" world. But his view—and the one I express, with trepidation, to fill in his gaps—is that data about the outside world processed by the I is even less reliable than what the I finds out about life through knowledge of the it. Especially when attempting to understand another being, we are at a disadvantage because of the very indirect access to another's it.

Groddeck makes a working assumption that the it, not external causes, brings about disease and injury. Philosophically, this stance is easy for him because it fits in beautifully with his vitalism, which refuses to see us as atoms determined by the material universe. If we grasp our life from within, we can determine the course of our life. Will and volition are allowed back into an understanding of the human condition. Vitalism makes it more probable that we can accept Groddeck's hypothesis about the internal cause of disease, especially the idea that we have a choice in the matter. The scientists that Groddeck disagreed with would see aggregates of people with diseases, judge what outside influences appeared to cause the diseases, and finally give pills or apply topical solutions to alleviate the symptoms. For such scientists, the patients were passive recipients of diseases. Groddeck, as a vitalist, anticipated the hypothesis of the existentialists who espouse choice and argue that we must center our life on decisions. The area of choice that Groddeck chose to work in was the area of illness and injury. He felt that through extended analysis of the it, we can more freely choose to be well.

His vitalist assumptions led him to the idea that we may choose to be well or ill, and his medical practice reinforced the notion that we have choice here. Much of his work was concerned with the methods of understanding and doing something about the it's propensity to make the organism ill. In existential terms, his practice was the means through which he clarified the options available to himself and to others.

Briefly looking at Groddeck as an existentialist helps to clarify the relationship between Groddeck's philosophy and psychology, but we must remember that Groddeck was a skeptical vitalist and hence a skeptic with respect to existential thought. If science tells us that our life is determined, Groddeck's thought tells us that the it determines our actions. The it, not our awareness, is sovereign. At times, Groddeck's vitalism seems to propel him toward the existentialists' view that we can choose our destiny—in Groddeck's sense to be well or ill—but for the most part, the it or its are great determined engines that create and manipulate the I. For my own use of Groddeck, I cling to the existential "fiction" of choice, but do so with modesty.

Groddeck does not deny that there are viruses and bacteria any more than he denies the existence of an outside world. These outside influences are at the service and disposal of the it. His philosophy inclines him to proceed in this way, and his psychology helps to clarify the choices that may be available to the organism.

We have to read Groddeck's works, suspend our materialist assumptions, work within his vitalist position, and phenomenologically test his ideas. In this way, we can appreciate Groddeck's ideas. But is not this too much to ask of people brought up in a culture dominated by science and not overly given to introspection? If we give ourself to his assumptions and see that the it is sovereign on matters of health and illness, the day-to-day consequences are obvious. Even though Groddeck sees limits to awareness, success through his assumption and methods does much to extend the frontiers of choice in existence. Death is a boundary condition of our existence, and even there we may find that we have more choice than we ever supposed.

Importance

Groddeck, as was stated earlier, tried as an I to find out more about the it, and he learned to bypass awareness in order to allow his it to speak more directly for the organism. To know thyself and to speak as thyself was a goal of utmost importance to Groddeck. In this section, we will discuss, first, some of the contents of the it, whether they be drives, structures, or patterns, and, second, some of the methods Groddeck used to get at what is important to the it. What makes both of these tasks difficult is Groddeck's relationship to Freud. He borrowed heavily from Freud in both description of contents and in method. He generously acknowledges these debts, but he rarely challenges Freud openly or elaborates his differences with Freud. This was an ingenious way to continue a friendship he needed, while avoiding those painful breaks others suffered with Freud. Freud would acknowledge their differences and lament that Groddeck would not enter the fold. Groddeck would gingerly avoid fractious disputes.

This strategy of Groddeck causes obvious difficulties for the biographer who must decide for himself the divergences between the two. It is as if Groddeck had a dual set of concepts to cover each situation. He might start off talking about the Oedipus complex, and by the time the essay was finished, the analysis was sufficient to stand without Freud's ideas. Groddeck's writings reflect his independence, his pluralistic approach to explanation, and his affection for Freud. Structures like the Oedipus complex are not of critical importance to Groddeck. Groddeck is more suggestive than systematic in describing the contents of the it.

For Groddeck, the it thinks in symbols. The associations that are made by the it may seem absurd to consciousness. For example, Groddeck did not like to go to performances of Richard

Wagner's *Ring of the Nibelungs* because the work disturbed him deeply. One day Groddeck understood that, for Wagner, the wife and mother were the same and that is the way Siegfried saw them. Now Groddeck began to understand the work and Siegfried's reactions as well as his own. The it can associate the wife with the mother in the way that the it can associate spatial arrangements within a synagogue with anatomy, or a sibling with an anthropomorphized animal in a fairy tale.

For Groddeck, the point of departure for analysis of illness is a symbolic gesture by the it. A sore throat may be a message from the it that a person does not want to speak; a headache may express an unwillingness to listen to something; a pain in the hip may represent a fear of bumping into someone undesirable. Empirically, a symbol may mean the same for one person as for another, or the same symbol may mean different things for different people. For example, readers may share the same rationale for a headache and have different reasons for a pain in the hip. Groddeck is not interested in collectives of people and generalization of symbols; he sees symbolizing by the it not only as a universal expression of humankind but also as a unique expression of each person and his or her it. The symbol is the it's way of expressing itself whether in dreams, illness, or in an everyday word or mannerism.

Freud spends only one chapter in his *Interpretation of Dreams* on the symbol, but Groddeck continually emphasizes the symbol. Even though the symbol seems so foolish at times to the I, we cannot ignore this way of speaking. The I may compare a penis to a building and quickly note the disanalogies. There are no qualifiers for the it. A building and a penis are one and the same. Since science and most discourse are written in the measured language of the I, a description of the it and it-talk sometimes appears ludicrous. This is an embarrassment that might have bothered Freud, but not Groddeck.

Groddeck also agrees with Freud on the primacy of sexuality in the organism. Groddeck, for example, ridicules the biologist's idea that sex is merely for reproduction. He spends several chapters in *The Book of the It* detailing the importance of masturbation in the individual's life. Masturbation starts before one begins to have intercourse and can be observed in the very old. We ride horses and rub our genitals in thousands of ways; mothers bathe their children and quiet them by sponging their genitals. For the individual, masturbation is a lifelong preoccupation.

Groddeck finds the Oedipus and castration complexes in analyses of himself as well as in his patients. His histories are laced with misunderstandings and adventures on these matters. Unlike those who fell away from Freud on this issue, Groddeck sided with Freud on the primacy of sexuality. Once again, however, Groddeck did differ somewhat with Freud. He demonstrates the importance of childhood sexuality, but he is not as tied to the hypothesis as Freud is. In many clinical examples, Groddeck does not link his analyses to sexuality, nor does he speak anywhere of sexual drives or motives. He finds sexuality to a great extent in the individual, but he posits no instinct or drive to explain sexuality and recognizes many motives other than sex to account for actions by an individual.

One of the things that endeared Groddeck to Freud was Groddeck's understanding that the fundamentals of psychoanalysis were association, transference, and repression. Groddeck made healthy use of these concepts. Groddeck, like Freud, concluded that every gesture, dream, or slip of the tongue was associated with the behavior of the organism. Groddeck suggests that the it makes these associations through symbols. Central to Groddeck's conribution is that organic illnesses are part of the associative network, not merely the result of external objects impinging on the organism.

Groddeck understood and borrowed the idea of transference from Freud. Although he did not write about the concept as extensively as Freud, especially with regard to its value in treatment, Groddeck was aware of the resistance in patients in a clinical situation due to transference. One of the ways he avoided this was to remain as unobtrusive as possible in the therapeutic situation. Finally, although Groddeck took account of resistence, he did not establish elaborate metaphors, like the censor, to explain what was happening. The I and the it are often in conflict, and the it, the governor, can keep secrets from the I. The

internal working of the I and the it is of less concern to Groddeck, the "pragmatist" who was more interested in consequences
of the it than in causes.

Groddeck makes use of symbol, association, transference,
resistence, and childhood sexuality; yet in his description of the
contents and workings of the it, he has certain emphases that
come from his own empirical work. His biographers always make
mention of his father, Schweninger, and Freud, all of whom were
important in his life. In his work, he pays homage to these
"fathers," yet seems able to reconcile his own views with theirs
and follows his own course. In his life and his patients' lives,
the stronger ties are to the mother. More important to Groddeck
in the Oedipus complex is the ambivalent bond to the mother
rather than the hatred of the father. In early chapters of *The Book
of the It,* he suggests that mother-love must be coupled with
mother-hate. The feelings are intense from mother to child and
vice versa. The resting point for the emotions of the child or
adult is the mother. We create the mother imago, the idealized
version of the mother that we bear in mind when we meet, love,
and betray others.

Although the intensity of the extremes of love and hate is
stronger towards the mother, these polarities dominate the way
the it conceptualizes all objects. The organism is ambivalent
towards all objects which are, after all, symbols and may be
variously interpreted. All symbols are, for Groddeck, male and
female, and we love and hate them. We rest uneasy in a world
where our ties to others and to physical objects are subject to
such ambivalence. An example of such ambivalence in sex roles
is the existence for the it of male pregnancies. Goiter, which
he cured in himself, and phlebitis, which he cured for Count
Keyserling, were examples of the it creating pregnancies in the
male. Finally, Groddeck spends much time speaking of birth
myths. We conceptualize birth before we can understand the
explanations given by others or are told the facts about conception. We may grow up with our it believing that birth takes place
through the mouth, navel, anus, or any one of many creative
solutions.

Groddeck is far less concerned with the precise contents of the it or the cause of these contents than is Freud. For Groddeck, the it is given, unknowable, and he does not try to conceptualize drives or forces. Early life and sexuality permeate the it; they are part of the it's historical legacy. Attachments to the mother, or lack of them, remain important contents of the it, as do the multiplicity of attitudes towards every symbol. Rather than the it having a drive of sexuality, power, or survival, the it is a repository of all these and other conflicting associations. Although the it is prior to the I, Groddeck does not speak in terms of instinct as opposed to learned associations. He retains Freud's language of repression, but in Groddeck's thought, the primitive forces of the it are not overlaid with the civilizing forces of the I. All the emotions and associations are in the it, and he does not say that some are inherited and others are only acquired.

In terms of contents, remember that Groddeck and Freud differ as to the basic structure of the organism. Groddeck's it, or life, incorporates the I and includes all action by the organism from conception onward. In his *Ego and the Id,* Freud called the it, the id. Freud's id is not nearly as inclusive as Groddeck's it. When we look at Groddeck's overall philosophical position, his vitalism, his bias against science, we can see how inevitable such a divergence was.

It is important not only to understand the contents of the it and the way the it works but also to discover how to gain access to the it. In Groddeck's terms, this means either for the I to understand the it better or for the I to subordinate itself to the it. In Freud's view, the primary avenue of access to the id is through the dream. The censor lets down his guard to allow unconscious material through; sometimes the material comes out as a compromise formation with conscious processes. According to Freud, free association is also a way to get access to the unconscious. In contrast, for Groddeck, the dream is purely secondary. And, he uses free association, or what he calls it-talk. His main avenue of access, however, is the symptom. The symptom was the starting point for Groddeck's analyses, and often his first question was, What are the purposes of this symptom? The symptom served a purpose for the patient because the symptom took him or her from a troubling situation and gave sympathy, power, surcease from guilt, or served many other purposes. Groddeck never settled on one purpose and always fell back on the idea that the it works mysteriously.

If the symptom is the point of access to the it, the I shows a resistance to the idea that the symptom has meaning. Sickness serves a purpose, and the I wishes to think its motives are pure. We resist the idea that we are manipulating others: we would never get sick to avoid going to a dance or just to receive sympathy from others! We also resist the idea, and perhaps this is most important, that we are not aware of all that we do. Ultimately, the idea is appealing that we can control disease. Yet when someone suggests that we are making ourselves ill, the conceited I finds this idea subversive. Moreover, we cannot accustom ourselves to the overkill of the it when we become very ill over a seemingly trivial issue. Why do we end up with ulcers when we do not want to visit our siblings, end up with a screaming headache just because we do not want to see blood? Why would we make ourselves sick just so we can see a doctor?

Once his patient had admitted that her or his illness was a bid for sympathy, the physical symptom became Groddeck's primary access to the patient's it. As he grew more sophisticated in analyzing himself, he saw any action or behavior as a point of access to the unconscious, the it. In the middle of his *Book of the It,* he begins a clever analysis of himself with the sensations he is having while he is sitting in a chair ready to write a letter. One nostril is slightly stuffed, and he is fiddling with his key chain and looking at what he thinks is Rembrandt's *Circumcision of Jesus.* He writes about forty pages on these associations and comes to great awareness of his life and circumstances.

As a physician, Groddeck felt his job was to deal with the complaint presented by the patient. Sometimes this treatment could take minutes and at other times it could last for years. Analysis of symptoms led him directly to their alleviation. By allowing the patient to free associate from any physical sensation, Groddeck learned about the person. He did not feel it was incumbent upon him as a physician to exhaustively follow all leads in patients. For him, cure was alleviation and prevention of recurrence of symptoms. In this way, he was less of an educator to others than he professed and more of a physician.

In line with this policy of cure was his choice of patients. Treatment of the chronically ill and dying constituted much of his practice. Although these patients were difficult and frustrating for other physicians, they provided Groddeck with some advantages. They were desperate for solutions, and their problems were not merely minor annoyances to themselves. Because they were desperately ill, such patients did not play their own games with him or resist his ideas.

Finally, Groddeck went from a style that resembled Schweninger's, where he gave authorative commands, to a much less directive approach. Transference still occurred, but Groddeck, according to his patients, hardly talked or interceded in the treatments; he felt that a person's it must treat itself.

Return

Groddeck returned from self-analysis to the world on his own terms with a great deal of knowledge about himself. He was an effective healer even though his interventions during treatments were far less frequent and intrusive than were those of other physicians. He had an arresting presence, for although he was five-feet-ten-inches tall, friends took him to be six-feet to six-feet-four-inches tall.

In this section on return, I will make little attempt to separate his personal from his professional life. Much that is said about his return applies to both. Fundamental to his return to others is that he wanted his it to relate to the others' its. As mentioned before, at times even Groddeck tried to put the it at the perusal and disposal of the I. His stance with others was to sidestep the I and let his it listen and subsequently talk. Ultimately, he wanted his patients to understand these principles and behave in the same manner.

Throughout his works, Groddeck describes ways of becoming more open and receptive to others. A cornerstone of his thinking is that we should return to being childlike but not childish. The child is open and receptive to ideas and not filled with judgments, prejudices, and fears. As he was fond of pointing out, the child only gradually becomes aware of the self, develops I-feelings. These I-feelings can get in the way of a genuine understanding of the world. The adult, in other words, is too dismissive of the information coming from within and without to have a good picture of the world.

As part of a childlike stance to the world, Groddeck encourages us to follow the Biblical injunction to "judge not, that ye be not judged." We spend much of life deciding what behavior is good or bad in others and how our neighbors stand up to these judgments. This leads to a great deal of guilt, blame, self-recrimination, and punishment, as well as revenge and anger. Although he does not explicitly make the tie, he implies that judging others leads to guilt and illness. If we are judgmental and not childlike, it is also difficult to allow the it to express itself or the I to have access to the it.

Groddeck's notion of tolerance is along the same lines as Nietzsche's critique of Judeo-Christian society. We do a great deal of harm to ourselves and others when we are judgmental. Groddeck's emphasis is, of course, on the harm that we do to the self. In his analysis, Groddeck anticipates the criticism of his views as amoral. He suggests that the child is amoral and we are better off in this position. Western culture has very deleterious effects on the individual. If Groddeck had called for revolution, he would have had to justify a society of childlike persons, although he probably would not have chosen to complete the task. At times he gives the case for them, arguing that beyond universal self-awareness would come tolerance for other viewpoints. All the ambiguities we see in culture—love and hate, violence and passivity, hubris and humility—would still be in the individual and hence society, but to be childlike would be to temper the extremes.

At one point Groddeck tries to quell the fears of those who would ask how the childlike would govern themselves; would the world be like Rousseau's idyllic or Hobbes's brutish state of nature? Groddeck suggests that we will never overcome the cultural propensity *to* judge others. Nor will we ever be free of the injunction *not to* judge others. Consequently, because of these opposing pressures, our institutions are not likely to fall apart.

Groddeck carries his quest to be childlike, or nonjudgmental, to analysis of specific sanctions and taboos we have developed in society. Every sanction we have masks a desire. There would be no need for norms and laws if the strong urge to do these activities did not exist. In much of his work, he uses the Ten Commandments to illustrate his ideas. For example, the Commandments tell us to honor our fathers and mothers. In Groddeck's analyses, he finds numerous examples of love of the mother and anger toward the father. Below the level of awareness, this father-hate may dominate the person. Groddeck does not let the mother off the hook either. He speaks of mother-hate as well as mother-love. The mother gives birth to the child and is then expected to care for the child. The child keeps the mother up all night with crying, keeps her (in modern times the father as well) tied to the house, unable to do much else. Society invents the nurturing instinct, and women cannot express animosity towards the child. Groddeck believes the mother's animosity toward the child exists and is reciprocated by the child. The injunction to love one's parents hides universal animosity that flows between parents and children. The same is true for the other injunctions; we are thieves and murderers, and we dislike our neighbors. Because the tendency to commit ourself to these actions is so strong, the taboos are also fundamental and strong.

The taboo against incest hides the child's love for the mother and the reciprocated love. He suggests that the taboo against onanism hides the basic propensity to masturbate. The story of Onan, Groddeck suggests, is the story of a protest against the law that made it mandatory to marry the wife of one's dead brother. Onan refused, casting his seed to the ground. This has become the justification for the taboos against masturbation while Groddeck feels that the violation of the law, refusing to marry a brother's widow, was the actual transgression.

As a cornerstone of his view on the individual, he notes that we are both male and female. His argument comes from conception where we are both sperm and egg. Society makes homosexuality taboo while we all have such propensities. Groddeck echoes Nietzsche's point that nothing human should be alien to us. Where there is a societal norm or a law, we are covering up universal propensities in human beings. Groddeck believes that society has become overly harsh in judging and that to "judge not" might provide some needed balance in the process.

The political consequences of Groddeck's stance seem remote to him, and he does not systematically derive them. The advantages for therapy, however, are obvious. If we do not sit in judgment, we are more likely to become acquainted with the it, which expresses all of our desired but socially unacceptable beliefs. We can sit in sympathy and listen to others if we judge not and accept all behavior as human. In his practice, Groddeck listened carefully to patients who protested too much. Those who hated homosexuals, reiterated how much they loved their parents, wanted murderers executed—they were, like the rest of us, homosexuals, parent haters, and murderers and had a particular problem with these desires. For Groddeck, to "protest too much" is to reveal a problem.

In his personal life, Groddeck tried to be nonjudgmental. He could not avoid the bind created by judging the nonjudgmental stance to be better than the judgmental one. He criticized the major religions for that propensity to judge. Yet he was tolerant of the intolerant; he was not going to pronounce the death knell for religion. He used the concept of "judge not" extensively, as well as the story of Christ, to help him with his analyses. All too human, he could not avoid judging, but he allowed judging to close out experience to him as little as possible.

When we return to the world as childlike, we unpeel the conceptions that the I has of the organism. We cast away illusions. We love and hate and desire to do what is prohibited by law and social norm. Part of this return is to understand our relationships to others. Groddeck suggests throughout his writing that our primary concern is with our own self. He did not become a doctor out of altruistic motives. In fact, it is best to understand the sadistic side of human nature that makes it easy for a doctor to inflict pain on others. Much like Nietzsche, Groddeck feels altruism simply masks selfishness.

Nowhere does he make the principle of selfishness known with more force than when he says that to mourn someone for more than three days is to mourn for our own self. Implicit in his view is that feelings we have for others are mediated by those fears, anxieties, and guilt we have about ourself. To overly love humanity or another being is, in a way, protesting too much. To understand this principle is to cast away another illusion.

Our realization of the primacy of selfishness has political, as well as societal, implications. We could take the position that this realization would bring out the Hobbesian man or the Thrasymachus in all of us. We could abandon all pretence of feeling for others and greatly increase societal competition and the potential of war of all against all. Groddeck's "selfishness," however, has other consequences. We do love others, although the emotion is definitely secondary to the care and attention we pay to ourself. We do not tend to become more ruthless once we realize that our it is preoccupied with our own plight. Understanding our own selfishness can make us more tolerant of others. Groddeck could have used Alexis de Tocqueville's concept "self-interest rightly understood" to show that we can then more accurately assess our relations to others. The notions of our own duty to and love of humanity is a false picture that, in Nietzsche's terms, brings *ressentiment* in behavior. According to Groddeck, our it understands our selfishness, and we should square our I with our it's view. Because of his views on prohibitions, Groddeck never felt that he could convince everyone to his view on human nature, so he never worked out the implications of the acceptance of his views by political institutions.

Groddeck's metamorphosis from one who gave authoritative commands to one who spoke infrequently to the other's it issued less from his concerns about freedom than from what effectively brought change. In this sense, he shared George Simmel's ideas on domination. Power is reciprocal, and to force a person to act is not the same as altering that person's belief. For Groddeck, the I might deceive itself to accept a command, but the it would not change. The it responds to metaphor, not command. In his nondirective way, Groddeck departed from many of the early psychoanalysts and resembles, among others, Carl Rogers, Rollo May, and George Weinberg.

Groddeck, as I have suggested, felt there were certain contents and specific organizing principles to be found in the it. Yet in his analyses, he did not constantly refer to only a few structures. This might very well be because his nondirective approach allowed his patients to discover structures for themselves. If you go looking for certain structures, you may find them, if for no other reason than to please the therapist. What is important to note here is that adherence to a rigid set of structures and careful theory of process can inhibit the strategies for curing. Groddeck's first preference was to cure illness; writing about the process seemed to be secondary. The openness of Groddeck as a physician worked to keep him from effecting closure on his views. He well understood this when he said that disciples would only make him hold his ground.

Before I proceed with the main body of this biography— a protracted essay on my elaboration of Groddeck's key concepts, my disagreements with him, and the future of this line of inquiry— I will attempt to make a few summary statements about Groddeck's philosophy, medical practice, and Groddeck himself.

Groddeck's skeptical vitalism is organized around the concept of the it. We are finite, conflictual beings with limited means to apprehend our own existence. That we die is a boundary condition of our existence, but Groddeck refuses to set the exact boundaries. Like some biologists of his time, he seems to harbor the suspicion that all men have been around since Adam. Death is also problematic because we are made up of its, not an it, and they are sometimes autonomous. When we die is dependent upon what we define as our being. Life might not cease with the cessation of awareness, or the I.

Fundamental to life is that the it decides how long we shall live. The it captures illness and decides when to be well. In Groddeck's most radical statement on the subject, he suggests that we die only when the it decides to die. Presumably, we are immortal if only we can stave off weariness of the it. For Groddeck, death—as it is for the deliberate suicide, or for the Eskimos and other communal groups whose elderly will their own death—is always a choice. Presumably we can live forever. Groddeck, in these ways, pushes on the boundary conditions of our life even more than the existentialists.

When it comes to realizing our freedom, Groddeck is far more pessimistic than the existentialists. We are lived by the it; the I may not have a great deal of choice when decisions are made by the organism. Here we come to understand why his views are conflictive. In matters of health as well as in other areas, the it and I may come in conflict. While the I might wish the organism to be well, the it can bring on illness. Conflict may come because the it works on truth, its associations follow one from another, whereas the I may be a temporizing, measuring, and rationalizing force. Finally, for Groddeck, conflict may be simply an illusion of the I, which thinks of the I in conflict with the it. What may actually be happening is that the it created and now controls the I. The I, however, tries to capture the workings of the it, of which the I is the child. Hubris is that the I thinks like a winner, but the it is ultimately triumphant.

Conflict is also manifest in the multiplicity of associations the it has of objects we come in contact with. We love and hate someone; we think of something as beautiful and ugly, right and wrong. We have a plural, conflictive view of the universe. For Groddeck, this richness of and openness to experience is truth. The I tries to simplify, or repress (in Groddeck's terms), the many and opposing views of the universe and clashes with the it's truth. Although Groddeck does not extend his argument this far, the implication is that the I simplifies reality at the expense of truth to enable us to act.

Our it is also in conflict with society. For the it, all things are permissible; for the I, many possibilities remain below awareness. In Groddeck's thought, society is restrictive, not helpfully civilizing as it was to Hobbes and Freud. In his work, he never deals with the revolutionary implications of his views by collectivizing the individual and supposing revolution; Groddeck sees the possibilities of a few individuals disposed to freeing themselves from society's sanctions. Even then, they would never be totally free. Mostly he speaks in terms of sexual liberation which for him does not seem to have great political implications. He has even less to say on violence and abrogation of the rights of others. There would always be conflict and misunderstanding between two or more individuals. We always feel we speak to another's I, not to his or her it. The realization of another's I is only partial understanding of that person. Groddeck believes the situation could be remedied somewhat if we would speak to each other's it. I have already discussed the difficulties in realizing this possibility.

Finally, it would appear that to be childlike would allow us to live as an it, be in harmony with other its, and control life and death. The child is in conflict with the universe because of his or her demand to be all powerful, to be the subject and not the object of the universe. The intercession of the I, of society, puts the it in a conflictive situation.

Life as manifest in the it is plural, conflictive, polytheistic, and given the limitations of the I, ungovernable. The it, not God or the individual, is sovereign for Groddeck.

Groddeck's medical practice was predicated on getting the it to choose health and life. The concepts Groddeck uses to conceptualize the contents of the it are often borrowed from Freud as are some of the methods of gaining access to the it. Rather than limiting the possibilities of what is in the it by pinning down instincts, complexes, and other contents, Groddeck prefers to leave the it as unfathomable and unknowable. In one sense, this choice brands him a mystic, but in a more formidable way, it allows the patient a freer hand in the exploration of the it. Freud's influence led Groddeck to posit structures like the Oedipus complex and the castration complex and to emphasize the importance of sexuality. Groddeck's own thoughts strain against closure and suggest far more possibilities.

Like most psychoanalysts, Groddeck is inclined at times in his work to generalize about the contents of the it to help others anticipate what they may find. But his counter tendency is to show through it-talk the infinite variety of associations that he and his patients made. The it-talk is almost an open invitation to find what you may in the it. People who read his works for the first time are often put off by his personal, varied, idiosyncratic associations. The initial response of a reader to these associations is that they cannot be true, which means the associations cannot be true for the reader. Groddeck uses the associations as illustrative of method; they cause the reader to develop his or her own it-talk from Groddeck's own rich associations and metaphors. What tends to mislead the reader is the impression that Groddeck, like most analysts, enjoys uncovering associations and complexes that are generally found in the its of many people. Hence, the tendency of the reader is to relate the associations to himself or herself and say true or false, instead of taking them as truth for Groddeck and as methodological training for the reader. The confusion is as much in Groddeck as in the reader. A person can read it-talk for structures and method because both are there. The influence of Freud led Groddeck, I believe, to structures, but I feel it is much more productive to read Groddeck as the rest of his philosophy inclines: as an invitation to open exploration of the it.

The scientist who tries to catalogue his ideas to ease the path of exploration for others is inclined differently from Groddeck. In his practice, Groddeck was concerned with consequences first. The idea was to cure the problem that presented itself. One could never be quite sure of why the cure was effected or, in Groddeck's terms, why the it decided to cure itself. His goal was much the same as in Jay Haley's family therapy: cure the presenting problem. Some problems were more intractable than others and led to a more complete exploration of life. Groddeck's goal as a physician was not the exploration of life. That was a luxury the physician could only indulge in with his or her own life.

I have only included a few details of Groddeck's life in these introductory remarks. Rarely have I tried to explain his life by his circumstances. Perhaps, without trying to ascertain cause, I might have shown a coincidence between his life and his work. Groddeck felt he rid himself of many illusions that he was a "good" human being. He was a doctor out of habit and accidental association, not out of a decision to do good for society. The Commandments blocked some of his strongest desires. He did not feel that his own ideas would lead to a better world. He saw real dangers in discipleship. He was self interested and believed that to mourn for or pity another was a form of self-pity. These illusions of the I, once dispelled, allowed him to live a life with less illusion.

Once stripped of these illusions, two choices remained for Groddeck: to live as Thrasymachus or Machiavelli's prince, giving full vent to the it, or to live, by cultivating awareness, free from bitterness, petulance, and fear. Groddeck chose to live in the latter mold. To Groddeck's admirers, this was evidence of a remarkable and deliberate transition. To him, however, this was not a heroic choice but merely the overwhelming direction of his it that, fortunately for him, was benign. For Groddeck, philosophy could only marginally improve one's life and circumstances. As with William James, one's philosophy was a matter of temperament.

A close examination of Groddeck's life, however, indicates a person who changed in impressive ways. He went from giving authoritative commands, as a disciple of Schweninger, to a nondirective healer; from a sickly to a healthy person; from a methodist physician to an open observer of life. By his own admission, he never fully understood or controlled his it. He never got over a chronic cough, a propensity to break up romances, and a tendency toward other foibles. Yet one has the feeling that he never despaired of doing so. Groddeck's life is testament to the idea that, despite what he says, to speak as the it or to control the it through the I is useful in making one's life governable.

Letters to B. J.

Dear B. J.,

I am flattered by your friendly disposition towards my work. Sometimes friends grow apart, but with us that is not the case.

Your piece in *Family Therapy* gave me a brief but perceptive glimpse into your thinking. The explicit sexual imagery, the frankness of your statements, and the tinge of irony let me see that you are still bold and at the same time modest towards your grasp of human existence—feelings I share. I must cease this line of discussion or all we will have in common is a mutual admiration society, and you will rightfully score me for being judgmental.

Recently, my thoughts have begun to focus on what I call the "Uncle Frank Syndrome." My mother's Uncle Frank had a curious habit. He would not drive a car until twenty minutes after he had eaten a meal. When pressed for an explanation, he would say it required twenty minutes to digest food before the head was clear. I have this wonderful mental image of the family grumbling and pacing the floor while Uncle Frank relaxed and peacefully visualized the progress of his noon meal, so that when the twenty minutes were up, the energies used to digest the food could be redirected to the road.

We can get a laugh from this, but only because, as usual, we are laughing at ourselves. I read that extended exercise is good for cardiovascular fitness, so I decided to run for one hour every other day. Why for an hour? Some people say twenty minutes a day is optimal, while others say one-half hour every other day is enough. My habit is no more justifiable than Uncle Frank's. I did not choose an hour a day on any scientific basis. As I look at the research of different doctors, I surely cannot be sanguine about choosing to run for an hour. And why run? Why not walk as others have suggested? Do aerobics? Do nothing, as George Bernard Shaw proposes?

What Uncle Frank and I have are generically called habits. They are laughable in that they have no sound basis in fact. They are not true or right; they are just regular. Yet as William James suggests, we could not exist without the habits that do not demand our full awareness. At the end of a day, we have tied our shoes, brushed our teeth a certain way, gotten sleepy and stopped working, put down a book, snacked at our favorite time, as well as indulged in hundreds of other habits. What makes my running and Uncle Frank's pause funny is that we have elevated them to ritual. Both of us have an awareness of doing these things and an awareness that we should carry them out. The ritual is one step above superstition, for Frank and I see some linkages to outcomes which can be explained pseudoscientifically. Uncle Frank will drive safely and I will improve cardiovascular health. We are a step above the superstitious who see the unknown powers interceding for them. Wear the same socks again and you will win the next game. Before we get smug again, the rituals and superstitions may all work because we visualize and have faith in the outcome. We differentiate ritual from habit, for the latter we keep less in awareness. When I tie my shoes I do so with a double knot. No longer do I actively remind myself that they will not become untied and that the tradeoff (looks better in a single knot) is well worth it in convenience.

As you see, I have begun thinking about habits and increasing my awareness of them. We tend to become smug about others who seem to be creatures of habit and social convention, while ignoring the fact that we are no different. We may decide our president's next action, fight our superiors, and then go home, eat our hearty third meal of the day (dessert last), and complacently sit in front of the TV to watch a favorite program.

I know, B. J., we were to be different. Electric minds. Irreverence. No habits. Yet we all slip into them. We are not Nathaniel Hawthorne's creatures who have no habits—we tend to have bowel movements at regular times or places, go for walks at the same time—I told you so. What can or need we do about it? I have taken to analyzing rituals and finding habits in the same way I look for illness. If we begin from Hawthorne's position that we might dispense with habits, why then do we repeat ourselves? For example, I always get tired at some point when reading and put down my book. When my eyes get "tired," I go do something else. The pseudoscience is that I tell myself I get fatigued, I get eyestrain. I can take this to mean that I should quit what I am doing whenever my eyes get tired. Why, then, can I read for hours, almost days on end, when I read certain things and yet need to quit immediately on others? My own experience indicates that fatigue is simply a convenient habit.

Here I go with my it-talk again. The same logic applies for reading and writing. At this point I was about to put down my letter to you out of fatigue. Why? Because I was beginning to doubt my powers of communication. Was I getting the point across? Most importantly, could not someone else get the point across better? Whenever I have these feelings of inferiority, I get fatigued. If I discover the source of fatigue, as in this instance, I can choose whether or not I want to go on writing. These feelings of inferiority bring on fatigue (the consequence) which allows me to go on to another activity and not compete with "superiors." Ever want to sleep all day when you were not up for doing certain activities?

These days I have begun to choose among some of my habits and to decide which to keep and which to change. In the past, I ate very little during the day. Sometimes I ate breakfast and skipped lunch. Other times I would snack in bits during the day. You probably remember my appetite as a runaway freight train. By three in the afternoon, the engine was heating up. From about twenty minutes before dinner until I went to bed, the engine got stoked. Then as now, I viewed the task of staying at an appropriate weight in the light of William James's idea of strengthening will. Abstinence, new diets, exercise—all are to maintain control. They are individually or in combination an example of James's idea of doing at least one strenuous activity a day to fortify will.

As you might have guessed, B. J., I have changed my strategy and now treat this identifiable habit of a runaway-freight-train appetite as amenable to change. In my self-analysis, I was curious about the late afternoon takeoff point, but it was not too difficult to figure out. Bored out of my mind at school, I looked forward to an afternoon snack. It was waiting at home as my reward. My sister was always on a diet; the cupboard was bare, so I had to forage. I always found something even if it was only social tea biscuits. Chocolate chips, the jackpot, were seldom available. Also very peculiar was my habit of starting to eat approximately twenty minutes before dinner, even though I knew a person could last without food for three weeks. In addition, I had always used the word *drunk* in connection with food. When I did my self-analysis, I began my associations at this point.

To make a long story short, while at my parents' home, I ate like crazy (curious phrase). At the dinner table, I would lower my head and do nothing but eat. In our family, my mother rewarded good eating by her approval, but to me, the most important reward for my behavior was that total involvement with food allowed me all the satisfaction of a good drunk. I did not have to hear what disputations were going on at the dinner table. Nor was I likely to be asked to take sides in them. My self-analysis revealed that I began eating before dinner so I could sit down in a partial stupor. Food to me was a drunk that I could not transcend.

Not surprisingly, I still overeat at parties when I am bored or uncomfortable, yet I eat sparingly when I am engrossed with what I am doing. (This is the first time the thought of eating has crossed my mind since I started writing—and it is now one minute after three in the afternoon.)

My wife has always treated dinner as the time when we can all get together and talk. Even now, this is when I space out. I simply do not hear my wife and kids. I think my foregoing analysis can help you understand my behavior at the table. If you recall, in the introduction to Groddeck's biography, I made the point that no situation or symbol is universal. Yet the social scientist in us looks for the generalization. In talking with my "critic-students," I find that for most people the dinner table is problematic. One extreme is a friend who as an adult takes her plate of food from the dinner table and eats in a different corner of the room.

Remember kidding me about my habit of rubbing my face, thumb and forefinger up and separated while rubbing my chin and upper lip? What were the consequences of this gesture? It covered the mole on my right upper lip. That is right, there is one there, and to me it looked as large as an elephant dropping. This habit was my way of covering it. That is why it is often hard to guess for others why they are doing some action. You did not see the mole, yet to me it was huge. What were _you_ covering up in those days by stance or gesture?

As you know, my daughter is best in the family at direct communication. Children and the elderly are quickest to bring to attention what concerns them. We in between resort to more indirect methods of communication. My daughter was sleeping an inordinate number of hours in the summer. My pre-Groddeck inclination would have been to see this as a response to the exhaustion from the school year, the tendency to take it easy. With my current disposition, however, I asked her what the consequences were of her sleeping. She answered, "I don't have to write thank-you notes to the grandparents." Without prompting, she went on to say that since her birthday four months earlier, every time she got the thought in her head of writing thank-you notes, she would become sleepy and go to bed. Faced with that information, she chose to do the task and was active again.

We have to become very careful about sleep and pseudo-science. When I sat down recently to write a book, I found myself very sleepy until I finally started writing. Sleep is a wonderful mechanism of avoidance. So is lack of sleep. Try to get to sleep before an important event. People say, "I was too excited to sleep" or "I was too nervous to sleep." My translation: "What a great excuse if I do badly; and on top of that, lack of sleep is like an anesthetic." But here I go again trying to generalize for others. The social scientist still lurks in me. We make generalizations all the time. Yet, as you know, whether the generalizations I make about symbols, symptoms, or habits are true or not matters little to the corpus of my ideas. Generalization is part of the social scientist's vanity. It is being the magician and, as the psychoanalyst George Weinberg says, trying to dazzle the patient—pure showmanship. I guess I (we) have been showing off for too long.

I will end on that note, for perhaps that is all writing is: showing off. Excuse me for unabashedly doing so, but I was so delighted to hear from you, apart from vanity, that I want to continue to engage your interest.

To our early freedoms and present awareness of habit, ritual, and superstition.

Augie Sayres

Dear B. J.,

I was happy to hear that my letter stimulated some thoughts about habits. You reminded me how it is difficult, even in speaking of habits, to get away from the idea of real or imagined physical discomfort or comfort. Fatigue, hunger, and even tying one's shoes are all linked with physical sensations that we may dream up or exaggerate. I was intrigued with your analysis of your occasional insomnia. Your mother had given you the remedy of Tylenol for lack of sleep. Ingenious of you to have trouble falling asleep when you argue with your mother on the phone. Then she intrudes into your thoughts, and you take her advice to make peace with her—you take the Tylenol. Do you still need to take the Tylenol? When I have gone that far in analyzing habits I find I have a choice. If you still have to take the Tylenol, then you might push back further into your past and see if this pattern of guilt and, subsequently, taking advice might have prior roots.

This brings up the question of how far back we must go to seek relief of our symptoms. I look to the future as well as the past to discover what events cause me concern. You are already aware of some of the ''deeper'' analyses that have worked, so I thought I might show you about provisional solutions that might also get results.

Before I left for England, I installed a new ceiling and repaneled our den. Aesthetically it was necessary (middle-class idea), but more importantly, I felt that something in that room gave me headaches. This was before I had met up with our friend Groddeck. When I returned from England and was no longer in the mood to put up with illness, I still got headaches in that room. In my self-analysis, as well as asking what the consequences of an illness are, I can also ask when and where it began. This helps me to answer the question of consequences. I got headaches when I watched sporting events. Yet there were times when I could watch them and not get headaches. The consequence of the headaches was that I would have to stop watching the events.

I began my associations and recalled a remark my grandfather made to my mother, which I heard second hand. He had seen me play in a basketball game and said, "I am amazed that Augie can run that fast. All I ever see is Augie on the couch watching TV." I cannot get back past that family story. My mother is a sports fan, and to my recollection (which may prove to be inaccurate), she never discouraged me from watching. Another memory I have is of my father telling me that a former captain of the Hempstead High School football team now drives a truck and that I, by implication, must think about a career and not just sports.

When I sit down again over this problem, I will begin with these recollections and the suspicion that my father or a male, not to my mother, laid the curse on me. If I progress further along these lines, I will tell you, but my purpose in this illustration is that we need not go back any further to alleviate discomfort. My first possibility would be to avoid sports on TV. Since that is as painful as my headache (after all these years I still am a Dodger fan), I pushed for a more agreeable solution. I found that if my wife or another female (my daughter) seemed angry with me, I would interpret this as anger about my watching TV. In all these instances, I would get a headache. My way out was to ask permission to watch a game: "Carole, does it bother you if I watch the Dodgers on TV?" Needless to say, no one wants to be put in the position I put Carole in. When I explained to her why I needed her approval, she reluctantly went along with it and I no longer get headaches. I will explore my problem further because the solution seems silly and awkward, and sometimes no one is around to give the "TV blessing." Also, as I have explained in my writings, we learn more about ourselves as we explore our life even if we do not cure our ills.

This analysis suggests why family therapists have had some success with organic illnesses. We need not go back to some traumatic occurrence or the precipitating event to find relief from symptoms. Altering present relationships or future concerns can intentionally or unintentionally alleviate them. A sudden interest

[margin note, handwritten:] If grandfather made the comment, why is it that female is where the permission needs to come from?

by my wife in sports, a broken TV, or a daughter who is a sports fan could prevent headaches.

In a more general sense, a cure of the fear of snakes can be avoidance. Like Groddeck, I see no need, other than our curiosity, for tracing an illness all the way back. He suggests that for certain ones, deep analysis is necessary. For me it is an empirical question. B. J., if you still have trouble sleeping, trace your illness back further.

This brings me to the catch-22 in which you entangled me in your last letter. You encouraged me to extend my analysis from illness to habit, and now you suggest that I may be criticized for aiding and abetting self-indulgent and, to use a clinical term, narcissistic behavior. I have partially answered the challenge by suggesting that only if we are curious do we have to go back further than is necessary for alleviation of symptoms. Groddeck related a wonderful story about treating a woman for a variety of ills. He sarcastically told her that she used her illness as an excuse to see a doctor. She did not show up for her next appointment. Twenty odd years later she wrote and told him that he had been correct and that she had never had to see a doctor again.

I would be toying with you if I said that this partial answer to treating illness is my final response to your challenge. Yes, you can alleviate symptoms through limited inquiry. As a physician, which I am not, I could stop here. Curiosity, however, gets the better of me and I must delve further into the solution. I cannot stop my thought at the point where my grandfather sees me transfixed on the couch. The philosopher in me says to dig deeper. I want to know as much as I can about myself and others to bring as much of the it as I can to awareness.

How then can I deal with the charge of narcissism? After all, Joseph Conrad is right in *The Heart of Darkness* when he suggests that we cannot always have our finger on our pulse. The answer is that I do not. No, I am not like the mystic who gives ontological priority to the inner world. Our inner and outer lives share in the goings on. Those who pay for conventional help may go inside for only an hour a day plus in dreams. I tend to tune in and out between activities and have not formalized the process. For me, the distinction between inner life and outer life is for convenience only. They interpenetrate: anxieties about tomorrow may lead me to childhood and back. If anything, functioning in the world takes priority, and increasing knowledge of the it gives me at least the illusion of being better prepared for the world. I know, cut the technical stuff. OK, what I am saying is that understanding the it helps me in my awareness of the world and of others. I have no intention of becoming a mystic and cutting my ties with the world

I imagine you are still not satisfied. You accept my pragmatic argument that increasing awareness will improve my communication with others and give me the choice of alleviating symptoms. But there lurks in your mind the cultural taboos against too much introspection. Regardless of whether or not the Greeks saw a navel as the center of the universe, in the United States there is a norm against over contemplation of one's navel. (Sorry to put words in your mouth. If I did not, then I would have to wait for your letter to respond. As intense as I am, I would make the following comments anyway.)

If I think of introspection as any thought about myself, then the taboo bears some merit. Indeed, most thoughts about myself tend to be judgments. I am better than the other person; he or she is better than I am; I am a poor swimmer; I am a good scholar; I am nasty; I am nice; I am fat; I am thin. In other words, most of what passes as introspection is merely a continuous self-judging contest. Joseph Heller in *Catch-22* captures this tendency we have. Colonel Cathcart is described as feeling great because he is only thirty-five and already a lieutenant colonel; yet he is already thirty-five and he is only a lieutenant colonel. We all play these introspective games. I am the best basketball player in my school; I am the best in camp; I will never make a pro. I shine over many of my contemporaries as a philosopher, yet I shrink from Plato or Sartre or our friend Groddeck.

Walker Percy is suggesting some of the same teachings when he speaks of the elusive self. This judging, continuous and relative to the objects we pick for comparison, can go on interminably and can be said to be time-consuming and wasteful. I can tell you to cut it out and be giving you good advice. Yet I know we still will do some of it. When I write an essay, I always question—as much as I try to suppress it—where my ideas stand in the pantheon. Surely examination of our friend Oedipus and sibling rivalry may make such self-comparisons subside, but they may never disappear.

If we practice introspection in the best sense, we can reduce self-comparisons. We can look at Zen and other Eastern disciplines as ways around self-comparisons. Also, my cultural criticisms, based on Tocqueville, try to show how, inevitably, majorities, who thrive upon distinctions, make comparisons which are unfavorable to minorities. If we eliminate self-judgments, we will increase our awareness of the it and make progress in communications directly with others, a more constructive introspection.

I leave you with these thoughts—from not the best or worst of correspondents but,

Augie

PS. Groddeck uses the concepts of the *I* and *it* while I substitute *awareness* and *life.* At some future time, I will go into the differences between his concepts and mine. For now, view them as synonymous and your analysis will not suffer a great deal.

Dear B. J.,

You are right. In my writing, I tantalize you with ideas about the self and I never follow up. My concern is with the problem of introspection and I never do indicate what the self is. As you know, I try to economize on the number of concepts I use to describe the structure of our existence. I have no inclination to champion the idea of the superego, the self, the Oedipus or the castration complex as universal. This is where we phenomenologists get into our greatest conflicts. Sure, in my own introspection, I use them and think of these metaphors as ways in which I record my past. I am careful not to generalize to the experience of others, however.

The self is one of many ways in which we may store our thoughts. Our it and awareness may treat this self or, if you like, selves, much as we try to differentiate our liver or our lungs as semiautonomous organs or systems. William James gives us an interesting description of the fluidity of what many people designate as the self. The self, as counterpoised to the I, or awareness, is composed of three components: the material self, the spiritual self, and the personal self. These selves, as he analytically breaks them down, may be more or less extensive for the individual: possessions as well as friends and ideas may literally be a part of our self; or in the limited view, we are only flesh and bone and inherited intelligence. We may puzzle at our urine, perspiration, and feces to determine the limits of the self. The self is entirely our construction much as are the pictures we form of physical objects and the supernatural. My interest in the self is the same as my interest in any constellation of perceptions we have. The self is a set of perceptions sometimes set in the it, sometimes set in the I, or awareness. The self is not a thing, but a description, much as others we have, constantly subject to plural evaluations. Much as we do with the heart

52

or the liver, we tend to treat this self as a sovereign entity with real properties. Here is where my real interest in the self lies. We treat this self much as we do other organs and we can scrutinize its ills in the same way. What are the consequences of feeling bad about one's self?

I am not suggesting the self is something real with properties that influence behavior; but much like perceptions of houses, trees, or bull horns, the self is an idea. As Walker Percy suggests and my example from Heller illustrates, this self (or selves) is designed by the it and/or I and suffers through much change and alteration. We may have one self, the many selves of a multiple personality, or a succession of selves like the protean man. In the last instance, the description of one's self may undergo complete transformation as one changes from revolutionary to ascetic to bureaucrat. The self is merely a way of organizing what others call him or her. The self is the container that we often wrap our other organs (sick or well) in. When we expect sympathy from others, it is this self that needs help. We make our legs, neck, or brain part of the self. The self has no necessary locus.

I am getting awfully academic and technical. Perhaps now I can show you that this creation called the self can also become ill. We constantly adjust our notion of the self; we feel incompetent, smart, expansive, powerless, rich, happy. We can begin our analyses with this adjusting internal picture of the self to treat our ills. Negative evaluations of the self imply a diseased self brought on by the it or awareness. The self in my scheme is decorative, a creation, not active. It is not the judge or the seat of judgment, but the verdict. From this verdict of the self, we can ask what the consequences of this verdict are. For example, if I decide I am stupid, I get others to overturn the verdict.

What I am doing here is reversing conventional wisdom on the self. One perspective usually wastes much time on an accurate description of the self which involves unending judging. The idea of self is turned into an evaluative process. What am I? Am I good or bad? These are moral judgments in which the self is compared favorably or unfavorably with the rest of the world. They can be greatly overdone. A more productive approach is the exploration of self as being, where we consider how extensive we are, what it means to be finite.

Any evaluative description of the self is the result of a decision by the it or awareness. These decisions are the most important for us to analyze for what they tell us. Any change in the self can be viewed as a communication to others. Hence, we can ask, Why are you feeling sorry for yourself, inferior, clumsy, etc.? Perhaps we can refine the question further from asking about the generalized self to asking about an organ or part of the body. In either case, we have access to our it.

B. J., perhaps all I have done here is to restate stoic doctrine in modern terms. As seen in stoic terms, the fault lies with thyself; in my terms, the concept of self is an indicator of what is actually wrong.

Augie

Letter to Dad

Dear Dad,

I am happy that you see some merit in my ideas on illness and philosophy and that you feel they may be broad enough to be of interest to others. My intention was to take the compliments and encouragement and continue easily with my work. Unfortunately, I feel compelled to tell you in detail how all this may apply to you. Since I got off the phone with you, I have been troubled by an expression you used with regard to something (I forgot the exact context) that had gotten on your nerves. You said it was a "pain in the neck." If that had been the first time you had used the expression, perhaps I would have let it slide. Yet I can remember that you have used this expression frequently. I could go so far as to venture a guess as to why and when you use the expression. If I did, I would be playing the role of doctor, not teacher; magician, not son. If you wish to pursue it, I will instruct you on how to follow up on this insight.

I am sure you can already see the linkage from what you know of my ideas on Groddeck and illness. It has probably been fifteen years now since you have known about the clogged artery in your neck. The it speaks in metaphors. It is no mere coincidence that the artery is clogged and something is always giving you a pain in the neck.

If I may anticipate what you will say: "It's a mere coincidence, a chance remark. How could there be any ties? It's true perhaps for others, but not for me." If you read some of my work or Groddeck's on the subject, you will see that people create illnesses that speak metaphorically. If we do not want to speak, *Shane* we may get a sore throat; if we do not want to run, we may twist a knee; if we do not want to hear, we may get an earache. Just the other day I heard of a case where a man applied for a teaching job in a public school and was hired. It is a job as a music teacher and the instrument the man plays is the saxaphone. With the job upcoming, he developed a badly swollen gland.

The position of this gland in the neck threatens a nerve, and he must undergo a delicate operation so as not to damage the nerve. Right! If the nerve is damaged, he may never play the instrument again. I do not know the fellow well enough to say if his it is going to prevent him from taking a job he does not want, if he will get into another profession entirely, or if there is yet another explanation.

I know you are skeptical. Coincidences? I have seen too many. A neighbor has shingles and admits to communicating badly with her husband. Not curious until you consider that he is a dermatologist. What better way to get sympathy than to present him with a disease to interest him. I have seen it over and over with relatives of physicians. We know the daughter of an orthopedic surgeon. She rarely gets your common cold or sore throat. It is always a broken bone, scoliosis, a separated shoulder. These are "real" problems and she has her father for consultation.

Another friend is married to a physician. She fully understood after some conversations with me that she presented her husband with assorted ailments. This came as an admission, not from my prodding, but from a reading of my friend Groddeck. She was in a class of mine and knew of my interests in illness and philosophy. Mrs. C came to me and said, "Last night I opened a window and pulled some muscles in my neck. The last time this happened I was stuck with this illness for eight months." I consider myself an educator and not a physician. Yet I realized that transference had occurred and I had become the substitute for the physician-husband. She had been speaking to me frequently before classes and believed herself to be a pain in the neck. Now she presented me with a pain in the neck. (Yes, transference occurs all the time between pupils and teachers.) When I realized what was happening, I said sharply to her, "Mrs. C, you can speak to me anytime. You don't have to bring me an illness to cure." What I was telling her was that she could speak directly with me. There was no need for her to think herself a pain in the neck and present it to me as a symptom for which I would have sympathy. Her pain subsided within the next few minutes.

I bombard you with examples. I am suggesting that I see too many "coincidences," too many tragedies. I invite you to look around to see in others, as I see, illnesses that are merely clever communications to others. This is a first step to understanding how the process works.

One last example and it involves me. I relate the story to show how ruthlessly we must apply the principles to our own self. After all, we can begin to see the process in others, and I guarantee that you will begin to see these connections, but for us individually, we keep insisting we have real illnesses. Not so! Let me tell you about the most difficult injury I had to analyze, one which was of overwhelming convenience. Remember that all illnesses are of utmost convenience at least on one level, below awareness. You may ask, Why do we want to endure pain? On the level of the it, the illness allows us to communicate to others and assuage our guilt or arouse sympathy in others. In my example, I suffered the pain of a sprained ankle and got sympathy, not humiliation.

I am sure you have not forgotten the high school championship basketball game against Levittown. Ike, our center, had begun to emerge as a star in the tournament. (I still grudgingly want to attribute his emergence to fortuitous circumstances and do not want to give him costar billing.) In the game, the other team's zone defense allowed Ike to shine, while preventing me and the other guards from scoring. So, I sprained my ankle in the first half and, consequently, played a miserable second half. See my motive—"Star Demoted"? No, the headline was to be "Star Injured (give him your sympathy)." I do not remember exactly how I sprained my ankle, but I found a way. Remember, it was the first time I had ever sprained my ankle. As the expression literally says, "I hurt myself." I found a way.

Why do I tell you this? You have to be ruthless with yourself. You cannot excuse illness or injury as due to some cause externa. Always look to yourself. Dad, you taught me that. There was a clear strain in your thinking that stressed responsibility. I simply carry it to illness. I remember the (by today's standards) cruel, but telling jokes about responsibility you used to relate every time we would evade responsibility: "You d-didn't hire me for the j-j-j-job b-b-b-because I am J-J-J-Jewish."

Your granddaughter Laurie went through the stages of seeing how others create their own ills, but she was loathe to give up the comfort of her own illness. As the supreme challenge, she asked me how the toothpick she had stepped on in the living room several years ago could have been anything but an accident. I asked her what she was doing at the time. After a pause, she answered her daunting inquiry herself without any prodding. Children and older people have an easier time making themselves aware of the contents of the it. She said, "I saw the toothpick there before I stepped on it. I could have avoided it." Then she went on to explain why she stepped on it. "I was younger and in the house with my friend Kraig. I felt guilty about being there with him alone. We were dancing. My foot found the toothpick." Of course, the injury took her out of the house and, for a child, out of a compromising position. The challenge: you are of the only living generation not to work such an analysis.

There are, then, two stages in understanding. First, you make empirical observations of others, and, second, you work on some illness or injury you have had. You need not begin with the pain in the neck, but you should try analysis on yourself after observing injury and illness in others. Like any kind of learning of this nature, you cannot understand or utilize it unless you experience it yourself. If you work an analysis on yourself, you will be hooked.

I hesitated before I wrote to you for I know how difficult it is for anyone to listen to another, especially one's child. After I got off the phone with you, I got a bad headache, and you guessed it, the locus was in the back of the neck. I felt guilty about not telling you of my theories. Once I recognized why I got the headache, it disappeared. Then I decided I would write to you and explain how the process works. Am I a good son? Am I altruistic? Do I want another headache? So I write.

What I see here is a general problem I now face. Everywhere I see people dramatically acting out illnesses. Several weeks ago, Carole and I went to a meeting at someone's house and saw a male acquaintance lying on the floor begging to be asked what was wrong. I accommodated. He had recently developed a bad back that had caused him great discomfort. Carole and I both noticed his demeanor was that of a child. Yet, he is ordinarily a calculating and careful practitioner of a staid and conservative profession. Coincidentally, his wife was leaving in a week to return to a position she held in another community two thousand miles away. They had come to our community for one year, and he had decided to remain. Disease is a good way to communicate to a loved one to stay close.

And here is yet another incident that demonstrates a connection between illness and a need to communicate. My favorite fiction writer was stricken with a disease, and I heard from others that he was terribly ill. When he recovered, this author stated that he would rather die than go through such an ordeal. Aroused by sympathy and curiosity, I searched for and found an article the author wrote about the Guillain-Barre syndrome from which he had suffered. He had come down with it around the time his wife left him.

It is difficult to make a long-distance analysis, yet my friends the stress theorists would hear me out on this one. Life-changes often precipitate illness. Where Groddeck and I have the advantage is that we go beyond the generalized idea of stress to try to find out why. Of course, the sufferer or would be sufferer is always the best judge provided he or she knows what to look for.

Garth Massey, a colleague of mine you have met, listened patiently to my ideas and could not see himself as internally causing his own illness. After a long pause, a sheepish grin crept over his face, and he blurted out that when he goes on his research trips to African nations he wills that he will not get sick. All I can do is leave him at this point to contemplate the full implications of his statement.

The most extreme and negative reaction I ever got was from a person who had read a few chapters in Groddeck's *Book of the It,* and when I asked him about his general impressions, with uncharacteristic violence he said, "This writing is shit! He is disgusting! It is immoral." Because his response was uncharacteristically strong, I suggested that with those very words he had begun to free associate. His immediate reply was that those words and feelings were always taboo for him, and he readily agreed to read on in Groddeck. Now he does wonderful analyses and has increased his awareness tremendously.

I am not sure how you will respond to all of this, but I feel compelled, whenever I see illnesses, to bring my ideas to people's awareness. Whatever your response is—This is awful! Not for me! Etc.—use your response (you will have formed one by now) as a point of access to increase your awareness. Perhaps this letter is a pain in the neck to read.

From one pain in the neck to another.
Love,

Augie

I Am My Own Mistake

by
August Sayres

Address to the Graduating Class

Spring Valley Medical School
Algonquin, New York

It gives me great pleasure to speak with future physicians and licensed practitioners about my ideas on philosophy, psychology, and illness. I come here as an educator, not as a physician, and I hope I can help you in some small way to develop a philosophy towards patients and practice. I expressed my debt of gratitude to the medical profession in *Will and Recovery,* which is my account of recovery from successful open-heart surgery. My purpose in that volume was to describe the relationship between doctor and patient and, thus, allow one to help the other. Today I wish to further address this concern.

First, I must acknowledge my great debt to my predecessor, Dr. Georg Groddeck. Those of you who are familiar with my work and that of Dr. Groddeck know that our claim is that the individual is the cause of all disease and accidents that befall him or her. Even language conveys this idea: we catch colds, we get pneumonia; our arm is not broken, we break it. Your first response to this idea should be negative. This idea seems to betray all you have learned about bacteria, viruses, epidemiology. What I propose is to give you Dr. Groddeck's justification of this radical hypothesis and conclude with some thoughts of my own.

Lawrence Durrell suggested that Groddeck never fully answered questions about epidemics nor was he ultimately interested in proving his hypothesis that we internally cause all our organic as well as psychological problems. What we need to do is search for the defenses Groddeck does set up for his idea. He suggests that his original contribution is to show that through the use of psychoanalysis we can extend the method of cure for neuroses to organic diseases. For Groddeck, an organic symptom, in much the same way as a symptom of neurosis, is a symbol of the it, or inner life, of the person. Groddeck adopts much of the baggage of psychoanalysis to show that symptoms of psychological and organic diseases serve useful functions for the individual. Although he does not refer to the history of medicine, his intention to dissolve the dualism between psychological and organic is much in the spirit of medicine as practiced until the end of the classical period and as described by Michel Foucault. The sore throat, as we label it today, was for the classical physician the red throat, fever, flailing about the bed, and constant attentions demanded by the patient. The headache was the pain, throbbing temples, ill temper, and inability to listen to what others are saying. Melancholia was described as lethargy, sluggish movements, persistent ignoring of outside stimuli, and inability to concentrate on more than one idea.

Dr. Groddeck was reticent to use labels like sore throat, headache, and melancholia, but not reluctant to treat all of these problems. Even in his time, advances were being made in establishing cause externa for syphillis, anthrax, and other diseases. He was not one to deny the existence of outside stimuli. His argument was that the individual, and more specifically his or her it, used or manipulated these outside causes to its own purpose. A person might break a leg to avoid running in a race, get a sore throat to avoid speaking, or catch a disease to atone for guilt. While Groddeck's analysis revealed his awareness of the cause externa, he always began with and relied on the cause interna.

To summarize, in the first part of Groddeck's argument (my reconstruction, for he nowhere deals with this problem systematically), he suggests that we may find cause interna in organic as well as psychological illnesses by borrowing the methods of psychoanalysis. Also, he appears to return to the classical definitions of illness to ultimately dissolve the distinction between psychological and organic. He uses this distinction only to indicate how much broader in scope his analyses are than those of conventional psychoanalysts.

At this point, I do not expect a swell of sympathy for Groddeck's and my views. Those of you open to these ideas will not want to give up training and knowledge about external causes and, at most, will give internal causes parity. For others, you see yourself in a war with Groddeck and other psychoanalysts. The struggle for primacy between internal and external cause, or psychological and organic cause, is a fight to the end. Psychological causes (cause interna) are merely causes where the intruding biological agent or chemical imbalance has not been found. It is only a matter of time until we control known organic diseases as well as soon-to-be-found-organic diseases like schizophrenia and depression. I could go on in this vein. It is not my purpose, however, to give comfort to your views, but rather to help Dr. Groddeck.

Another argument Groddeck gives is empirical. In the cases he details, finding the internal cause leads to cure or prevention of an illness. A preponderance of empirical data indicates that he had great success with treating what you would call organic illness. His practice was based on many terminally ill patients who were referred to him by other physicians. He had a fine reputation and strong following. Groddeck's data is impressive if we read through his books and clinical communications. But positive data like this tends to fade under the glare of data from physicians and related professionals who report clinical and experimental success. Unfortunately, we often fall victim to majority views when what we are after is truth. I will comment later on this data.

Groddeck never *stated* his hypothesis as a law, but, instead, viewed it as a working hypothesis. It was but the starting point for him. In the early years of his practice, he was under the influence of Schweninger, Bismarck's physician, who trained him in treatments that employed diet, baths, and authoritative commands. Through his own practice, independent of Freud, he began to see the important role the individual (or his or her *it*) plays in selecting disease in response to problems of living. He overturned the assumptions of his early training and took up as a working hypothesis that organic illnesses are caused by the mysterious forces of the it. This was his operating assumption, just as yours is to begin with cause externa.

At times, however, Groddeck did *treat* the hypothesis as law. When he writes about his practice as a wartime physician, he takes the position that some of his patients actually, in our modern slang, bit the bullet—walked into a line of fire, acted clumsily or stupidly so as to jeopardize their lives. But for the most part, he was content to treat his hypothesis as just that. The position he ultimately took was that he as a physician operated under this assumption, his patients believed him, and the world and science be damned.

I could stop here under the premise that you would read this lone voice and take his ideas seriously, as a leavening to your own approach. Two problems make me continue. First is the difficulty of reading his ideas in the appropriate spirit because, among other things, he discourages followers. This I have dealt with in my book, *Georg Groddeck: A Biography.* Second, I believe I can strengthen his argument and propel you to a serious consideration of his ideas.

Groddeck made the point that there is no real difference between the treatment of organic and psychological diseases. We find that now the medical profession is beginning to accept a broader definition of disease and, therefore, health. Several years ago my talk would have fallen on deaf ears. Medical practice resembled the practice of methodists in the early Roman empire when they would isolate a symptom, name it, and experiment until they found something that relieved it. Probably none of you is willing to go as far as Dr. Groddeck, but today you are at least open to ideas that stress, diet, and environmental factors do contribute to the cause and cure of disease. The work on stress of Hans Selye and his followers has given you the possibilities of convergence with those who treat the mind. The work on biofeedback of Barbara Brown and her colleages is another linkage to those who see mind and body as influential in the development of disease.

It is no longer difficult to accept the fact that disease may have a cause interna that contributes to its development. Allergies may be worsened by stress; flu or strep throat may occur after a loss in the family, a disappointing vacation, a troubling anniversary, or a change of job. From the point of view of therapy, this knowledge does not change most treatments or preventive programs. Some practitioners may perceptively see the linkage between stress and illness and ask patients to reconsider some life circumstance. As my own physician has told me, he wishes he had hours to speak with each patient, for he believes profoundly in cause interna. The demands of time and the comfortable habits of the past, as well as the convenience of pharmaceuticals, make it easy to sink back into methodist treatment.

If the conveniences of practice do not lead to change in treatment, the medical practitioner does not have much impetus to change. Even if you, as physicians, accepted Groddeck's argument, you could use methodist treatment and justify it in the following way: even if all causes are interna, a physician can relieve all symptoms by attacking the cause externa that the patient has latched onto. There is a good deal of comfort and truth in this view—truth, because regardless of the cause, you can cure a sore throat using pharmaceuticals.

Psychoanalysis is sometimes slow and uncertain, and current methodist treatment is swift and certain. You do not need the cause (interna, in Groddeck's sense) to work the cure. Most of you are comfortable with methodist techniques because almost all of you have been trained in them, have much time invested in your training, and have already developed rivalries with your few colleagues who have chosen psychiatry.

Even if you have reversed causality in your mind and agree with Dr. Groddeck that the it causes disease, you may continue to cling exclusively to the treatments you have learned so well. I come here not to convince you to give up all of that, but to suggest that you begin with Groddeck's assumption and use medicines as a last resort. This is a wish, a dream on my part, but I will be satisfied if only a few of you alter your ways. Your teachers who have practiced for many years can attest to their frustration in dealing with patients with chronic complaints. No sooner has such a patient recovered from a sore throat, laryngitis, and so forth, than the symptoms recur. Before we knew about Groddeck's ideas, we could classify patients as either hypochondriacs or real patients. This distinction, however, did not stop the flow of people with problems coming to doctors. Like the paranoid who may indeed have real enemies, the hypochondriac may indeed have a sore throat, an ulcer, or eczema. You, the physician, must treat him, and he will not take kindly to any suggestion that he is deluding you. In other words, our pharmaceutical weapons cure. However, they do little to prevent recurrence. This dilemma frustrates the physician who becomes a partner in a damage-control routine.

I believe I have given you reason to seriously consider Dr. Groddeck's thoughts about a cause interna, but I have not yet given you a sufficient one to prompt you to alter your practice. That will come later, but first I would like to consider Dr. Groddeck's justification of his hypothesis on the basis of empirical data. In four books and numerous articles, Groddeck documents his successes with patients. I suggest that he was fifty years ahead of his time. His fellow scientists are just now doing studies confirming the relationship between stress and organic diseases. Groddeck is, however, still ahead of his colleagues because his work indicates specifically how to treat and prevent disease. The proponents of stress theory may conclude that people should avoid difficult job changes, taxing vacations, and so forth; and this is sound advice. But Groddeck viewed the causes of illness as much more specific to the individual: it might be that her new boss reminds her of her father, or his vacation causes him insecurity because he is less able to provide protection for his wife on a superhighway than in their home.

In the libraries, the evidence for success with empirical methods of curing organic diseases overwhelms my writings and those of Dr. Groddeck. The chances are you have been exposed little to either of us, other than the articles Dean Bowerman so kindly distributed to you, at my request, as a preliminary to this talk. As I suggested earlier, let me emphasize that proof of one method of cure is not proof that the other method is wrong. You could accept both ideas. Also, the method of proof differs. Data for our hypothesis are not only empirical but also what I call phenomenological. You are familiar with the empirical data. In my article "Observing Illness in Others," I point out how one first becomes convinced of the cause interna by careful observation of others. As physicians, you are in an excellent position to ask questions and follow the history of a patient. If you allow yourself to see disease as a form of self-expression, not isolated from other human behavior, you will become convinced of the importance of the hypothesis. Phenomenologically, you will then be prepared to do a similar analysis on your own medical history. Once you do these analyses, you may change your ways of practicing medicine.

What I am suggesting here is a different way of evaluating evidence. Heretofore, you have had mentors who have served up conventional wisdom and sometimes extraordinary insight into disease and its causes. Ultimately, you are the evaluators of this information, and practice gives you a whole new body of data to work from. All I am suggesting is that you take a careful look at your patients, as well as at friends and acquaintances, and see if you can find more about the cause interna. We could argue ad infinitum as to whether we literally catch disease. As Freud understood so well, each of us must test these hypotheses on ourself for ourself. How can we argue that there is no such thing as the Oedipus complex or that Freud exaggerated the importance of childhood sexuality unless we turn to ourself for data? Freud used himself as a source of data, thought of himself as a scientist, and yet worried about "objective" verification of his theory. Concern about objectivity is proper, yet it is unwise to slight the phenomenological basis of much of our data gathering. "Know thyself" is a good starting point for understanding disease as well as any human behavior. Before you dismiss Groddeck or me, ask yourself in the way suggested by my article whether your own illnesses have metaphorical meaning.

Earlier in this talk I stated that Groddeck's hypothesis was a working hypothesis. In his practice, he began with that idea and ultimately defended the effectiveness of his hypothesis by pointing out that he and his patients believed in it and that as a consequence he was successful with cures. I will expand on the hypothesis for you—more than he ever cared to—and suggest what its implications are.

Let me show what happens if we begin by giving no particular priority to his hypothesis. After this talk, you may confer some status upon Groddeck's hypothesis, perhaps even make it coequal with empirical methods of cure. In other words, you will grant that *some* organic illnesses are caused by the it. If, however, we use the word *some* in the hypothesis, then we begin to excuse *all* illnesses from being caused by the workings of the it. Why is there this tendency? Because below the level of awareness, we are creating illnesses that are helping us out. We may be enduring pain, even endangering our life, but we get out of going to parties because of stomachaches, are permitted to stay home and write because we are ill enough to collect disability pay, or develop headaches because we do not want to listen to our spouse. Illness is a wonderful excuse, and on top of it all, we get sympathy for using this excuse.

Because we try to create a positive image of ourself, we have difficulty admitting to our own self as well as to others that we become ill to avoid facing problems or to get our own way. Thus, if we use the word *some* in the hypothesis, we will tend to look upon the avoidance behavior in ourself and others as genuine and blame *all* ill health on cause externa. At this point, the hypothesis becomes worthless in practice, a mere idea for amusement and curiosity.

My justification of the working hypothesis that *all* organic diseases and accidents are caused by the it is a pragmatic and existential one. In practice, if we do not begin with this hypothesis, individual resistance to the idea is so great as to render it useless. Still, can we turn around and claim the status of a law for the hypothesis? My justification runs in a slightly different fashion from Groddeck's, one in fact that might have struck Groddeck as putting too much stock in the *I* , or *awareness* (my term) and too little in the *it,* or *life* (again, my term). We are trying to develop *character* in the world, to seek *integrity,* to gain our own sense of *importance,* and to *return* to the world on our own terms. We should try to capture our life from our own it and from others. Groddeck's hypothesis, a working hypothesis, gives us the possibilities of winning back more of our existence. We should decide whether we are to be ill or to be well, whether we are to communicate to others directly or through guile. If we do not accept this hypothesis, then we are relinquishing a certain hold on existence. Another way of viewing this is that Groddeck's working hypothesis is a postulate, for existentialists, of Sartre's hypothesis of the importance of choice for individuals. If I lift Sartre's hypothesis to sovereignty, I carry Groddeck's hypothesis with it.

Now that I have stated the hypothesis in my terms, I will settle in to analyze some problems that might be occurring to you. No more than Groddeck believed do I believe that we can be immortal or that we can ever be "well." The human condition is to be involved with this heroic struggle of awareness to gain preeminence over and above life. I prefer, whenever possible, to control rather than be controlled by existence, even if this ultimately is a myth. If in the long run Groddeck is correct and the I is merely a tool of the it, a creation of the it, I take the chance of being a dupe. If possible, we make decisions based on our I and do not defer to the it of others. Groddeck's working hypothesis is for me a stance towards life, an outlook towards existence. In analyzing the lives of others as well as my own, I find enough evidence to suggest that with work we can regain some control over life, especially with respect to illness.

One of the questions that must come to you is what happens if you cannot find the cause of illness in yourself or others? If I have a headache and take an aspirin, the pain disappears, but the headache is likely to recur. I would, therefore, rather endure the pain of the headache in order to unearth the causes of the pain. Cured or not, I am richer in terms of awareness. But for you, as physicians, faced with this situation as individuals or with patients, I am not recommending that you forget about empirical cures. At a certain point, pain becomes unendurable or threatens health permanently. You must then administer the classic cures.

Perhaps my recent home improvement may serve as a metaphor. I installed a new medicine cabinet in my bathroom, one smaller in capacity than the earlier one. I had to decide which medicines would no longer serve as a crutch. I saved only ones I might need in an emergency. The cabinet, although smaller, is still there, stocked with a minimum of remedies; and I have not discarded my doctor's telephone number, insulted my pharmacist, or forsworn the advice of others. But I am the initial resource in the understanding of my illness, as you should teach your patients to be in theirs. The existence of the medicine cabinet as a backup is to keep us from fanaticism and for an emergency when we do not have the time or self-access to solve our problems immediately.

What I am advocating for you is not a new hypothesis about illness, but a radical change for many of you in your stance towards existence. Your present role, as prescribed for you, is as a savior. Patients come to you for answers to their problems and you apply the salve or lotion. They may be able to function again but are no further along in terms of awareness than they were when they came to see you. They are grateful for your wisdom and further in your debt. The situation is not unlike the teacher who lectures to provide answers for a test. The student has answers, perhaps respects the teacher, but does not know what the questions are. Dependency, and not character, has been fostered.

To practice medicine with the hypothesis that illness is a metaphor created by the it takes an extreme turn of mind for it to be successful. Luckily, as I have illustrated with the metaphor of the bathroom cabinet, it requires no abandonment of the empirical methods you have learned so well. What it does mean is a radical reorientation to those you call patients and the need to make them more than coequal in knowledge of themselves and their circumstances.

Thank you for your time and your attention. Good luck in your careers. I wish you and your student-patients "well," in my sense of the word.

Letters to B. J.

Dear B. J.

I had a very interesting encounter with illness last night. I was reading Nikos Kazantzakis's autobiographical work, *Report to Greco,* when I became dizzy and nauseous. My right ear hurt and this seemed to be the locus of my problem. The room and the book were weaving and spinning. I tried to read more, but could only proceed line by line. Quickly dinner came, and I fought the urge to lie down and sleep. Nausea made it difficult to eat, but I forced myself, refusing to give in to the malady. I ate two grillers (soy hamburgers I smothered with raw onions) which were of my own choosing; the rest of the family had hamburgers. With relish (no pun, just association), I overdosed on broccoli. Finally, I ate only one half of a delicious yam.

At this point you are probably about to throw down this letter, finding my description of dinner as boring as Franz Kafka's letter to his sister telling her what he planted in his garden. All is to a purpose, however. Our it makes choices and decisions, and when I sat thinking of the dinner, several associations came up. In the past, I had felt that onions and broccoli would upset my stomach. Already feeling like Jimmy Stewart in *Vertigo,* I doubled my problem by trying to gorge myself on foods that would have, in the past, compounded my discomfort. When I ate the sweet potato, I remember thinking how exceptional it was. The inside was soft and sweet, yet not overly ripe. As I thought about it, my daughter had told Carole she would not eat one for dinner. Since sweet potatoes were the cornerstone of the meal—Carole had gotten a great urge for sweet potatoes— she was angry that our daughter would not eat them. I must have been angry with Carole because I complicated things by eating only one half. Do not picture in your mind a drama of a wife yelling at her daughter and her husband for not eating their sweet potatoes. All this is nuance. Moreover, none of these perceptions needs to be true from the standpoint of the other participants.

For me, however, as I look back at the incident, free associate about it, this is what I see. I saw the meal as an attempt to aggravate my wife and make myself sicker.

I sat on the couch after dinner trying to will through my discomfort. The angle at which I sat expressed my vertigo, for my body was at forty-five degrees with the couch. My wife was reading, and as I think about it, by remaining in the room, I was inviting further comment on my illness. I had told her it was nothing serious; I was just a little dizzy. She looked at me and said, "Augie, you ought to go in and lie down." I grinned at the suggestion and was about to get up, when I realized that lying down was the consequence I wanted from my vertigo. Mostly through body language I conveyed to my wife that I wanted to lie down. At that point, I refused to give in to my it, and I told her I would walk around the block and think my way through the vertigo.

As my own analyst, I have a great deal of freedom. I have no need to wait for an appointment to have someone help me think this through. An alternative would have been to sit in a quiet place and free associate about this illness. I resisted, for I had meditated several times that day (another part of the story), and I fought the idea of further rest. The opposite is to be physically active and I chose to walk. While walking or jogging, one can take time and place for granted, and associations can flow easily—just as they can when one is quiescent. I jumped a mile when Carole rode by on a bike sometime later (five or forty laps around the block) and asked me how I was.

As I look back at the walk, the technique I was using was similar to what George Weinburg calls the hunger response. If you deprive yourself of what you want (in this case rest), then free association brings up useful information. What immediately became obvious was that I had tried to force myself to bed all day long. I had awakened at my normal hour of 6 A.M. and prepared for my run at 8 A.M. There was nothing unusual about this as I run for an hour every other day, and for the last month I have begun at 8 A.M. (I had gone to bed earlier than usual.) I meditated for forty minutes after exercising because I felt I might be tired during the day. During my run, the unusual happened. My partner and I found ourselves ahead of schedule. We were setting a record. He runs twenty minutes, and I join him in the run for forty minutes to his house and then amble home for the last twenty. As you know, we run for time and do not race. On this day, I could have let up when I got to his house, but I pushed and ran faster than I ever do. All the time, I was thinking how tired I would be during the day. Also, I thought of how stepping up a normal pace can cause people to be dizzy when they get up from sitting later in the day. I was in an ongoing debate with myself: I told myself that I was not running that much faster and, besides, I do not get vertigo from standing up quickly; yet I felt the results of the run would be dizziness and fatigue.

Later in the day, we began an hour's journey to pick up my twenty-two-year-old son from the hospital where he had had his tonsils out. As you know, B. J., he lives in New York and was here for a visit. He had asked his mother to make the appointment to have his tonsils out during the vacation. More about this shortly. The day was hot, and my wife had the car window open only a bit and asked me to open fully the window on my side. I was aware of the wind's impact on my ear. Annoyed, I closed my window and turned on the air conditioner.

As you are familiar with analysis, you know the importance of the day's events in interpretation of dreams. So it is with illness. As I walked around the block, the day's agenda came into view. It was not my regular agenda—doing normal exercise, visiting up my son, coming home to mow the lawn, and grading papers—as I had carefully planned. No. I was trying to get an inner-ear infection and lie in bed for a few days. This became obvious as the associations flowed: from meditating when I arose to sticking a hard instrument in my ear to clear away the wax shortly before I became dizzy. This was not the first time I pulled such a trick and caught vertigo. I did so in my pre-Groddeck days and was laid up for the better part of a week with doctors, medicine, sympathy—the whole works.

It seems odd to me, too, that below awareness we are hatching plots, making plans that seem to have little to do with the ostensively important events of the day. When I go into my *reveries* I find this time and again. Sure, I go to work, meet with X and Y, go out to dinner, and read for a bit afterward. Yet the day may have been hatched on a chance remark someone made that I took as an insult, a conversation overheard that caused me to worry about my taxes, the broken fan belt on the car, or scab on my cut. Try to muse about your day and see what you come up with. Exercises like this changed me from the smug existentialist extolling consciousness and choice to one who begins with an existentialist's stance but is no longer so certain about his choices. More about this change later. Now I wish to continue my it-talk.

I needed no convincing that I had worked hard to cause the symptoms of nausea and dizziness. There was my initial feeling that this disease was caused externally, but these delusions no longer last. I cannot fool myself anymore into thinking exclusively in terms of cause externa. The more serious resistance comes from thinking that my illness, in this case vertigo, will prevent me from interpreting my illness. The initial impetus is to suffer through the disease. How can one think with dizziness or, on other occasions, a headache, a head clouded with fever, or an excruciating pain in the rib cage. This is a resistance one must fight, for below the level of awareness, rest is being prescribed, or some other change in behavior, and the tendency is to go along with it. On the level of awareness, few want to be sick. Beware then the comfortable feeling that *this time* I will just ride the illness through.

I had a difficult time in that last paragraph. Notice what a strange example I gave, "an excruciating pain in the rib cage." I thought first of an ankle sprain or a torn calf muscle, but I rejected them. If I give these examples, I may be creating possibilities of injuries for myself in the future. In the past, the ankle and calf have been "weak" points. It makes no sense to give myself the suggestion. My it, and I assume the it of others, is very creative.

A few years ago, after heart surgery, I found myself getting weaker by the day. This weakness was inexplicable, but I tried through will (the conflict between life and awareness) to see my way through it. What suddenly occurred to me was that I was playing this scenario the way John Wayne would. In a flash, I saw that this was the way John Wayne acted in a film I had just seen in which he was slowly dying of cancer. What I had done was to re-create the role played by Wayne in the movie. If I am ill, one of the things I do is to see if I am not acting out some illness or injury that I read about, saw on film or TV, or heard from a friend. Real life instances, in this way, can be contagious. Of course, the same holds for giving in to an epidemic. The flu is going around so I will catch it; everyone seems to be getting the twenty-four-hour virus.

In the case of my John Wayne syndrome, I never did analyze why I wanted to fade slowly from existence, or at other times why I want to succumb to an epidemic. Maybe I am envious of the sympathy the victims are getting. Perhaps the strain of warding off the disease seems less inviting than the bed rest offered by the disease, than even the ultimate rest it may offer. The it continually amazes me at how clever it is.

I know. Get on with it. The John Wayne incident is interesting, but what has it to do with the vertigo? Probably nothing, maybe all. When you ask me to trace my thoughts on an illness, I show you how my mind takes flight and I let it go. It-talk is personal, idiosyncratic, and the way one begins to make important associations. Groddeck's *Book of the It* is filled with such talk. He never tells what it-talk is supposed to do for the reader. What reading the book did for me was to inspire me to engage in it-talk. I hope my it-talk inspires you to it-talk. Maybe John Wayne, rib cages, air conditioning, sweet potatoes, or vertigo will trigger associations in you; or more likely other words will act upon your it. Poets and writers whose works are rich in metaphor, and specifically Kazantzakis (as I will show you in this vertigo case), trigger—as do the walk, the dark quiet room, or the psychiatrist's couch—a rich set of associations.

The John Wayne syndrome is not as irrelevant for me as it seems. My vertigo was an attempt to suffer the same consequences as my son who was trying to recover from his operation. Vertigo was a case of imitation in the same sense that I picked up the Wayne syndrome. In the same way as my son, I wished to recover from disease by rest.

Now that I have neatly tied this letter together through association, no doubt you are sifting through the rest of the letter to see if there is enough evidence for a conclusion to my example. Am I closing this letter because I am running out of time to write today or, more likely, is it my propensity to think and write in terms of suspense? After all, social science is an unveiling for me, the uncovering of mystery. Why should I not write it as I experience it. I am not ashamed to say it: devouring the Hardy Boys series was my first comprehensive study of style. It suited me and still does.

Nonetheless, you might anticipate through my associations where I am going. We inevitably make studied guesses when we observe the associations of others. Sometimes we can guess correctly. More often we ourselves remain sovereign over our strange and wonderful associations.

My next letter is soon to follow. Stay on the edge of your chair.

Augie

PS. If you begin to suffer from symptoms of vertigo, you know where you caught it.

Dear B. J.

I will continue with my analysis of my vertigo. When we were leaving the hospital after visiting my son, I was somewhat depressed. Carole and I felt his attitude was poor and he was doing little to help himself. In dramatic fashion I said, "You know, sometimes I think it would be easier all around if he didn't survive." On the way home from the hospital, I chose a new mantra to meditate with, "judge not." (I had been using the same one, "character," for a month.) I took on Groddeck's phrase because I had felt so guilty about judging my son. All of these choices were below the level of awareness. During my self-analysis as soon as I remembered making that statement, I knew where the origin of the vertigo was.

As with the John Wayne syndrome I once caught, I wanted the same consequences for myself that my son was experiencing. Vertigo, as I experienced it, left me with the overwhelming need to lie down and act in a pathetic manner. These were thoughts about what I deserved and what my son should be doing. I recall several times thinking that he should be lying down more.

As I continued to walk around the block, I began to free associate about my son and my feelings. He was actually not behaving badly, and my statement was not objectively about him, but about me and my anger and guilt. Often I find that my feelings about others are projective. As Groddeck would say, "We protest too much." What we hate, feel intensely about, avoid—these are most often reflections about our own self. Now you can see why I can print in a letter what I said about my son. The quote was about me and not him. I remembered my trip to camp as a child. Instead of going with the rest of the campers, I was late and went on a train by myself. While riding on the train to a summer camp when I was much older, I recalled the younger Augie fearing the camp, not knowing anyone. I remembered the picture of myself as a child with a beauty mark on my upper lip. Yes, the infamous one that causes me so much grief. Perhaps it is a metaphor for the importance of aspects of our life which are of no importance to anyone else. It is the idea below awareness that dominates our existence.

My mind flashed to the nurse in the hospital who was very overweight. At the time, I was amazed that what dominated her was a beauty mark on her neck. Quickly I got a picture of a man in a TV movie with a scar on his face. The movie was playing in my son's room and we were casually looking at it. In this old Jerry Lewis comedy, Jerry was being browbeaten by the man with the scar. The scar on this gangster ran from the outside edge of his nostril to the corner of his mouth. You guessed it. For me, it looked as if he had gotten the beauty mark removed.

My mind went deliberately to prior thoughts on the beauty mark—interpretive work leaves threads hanging all over the place. I picked up the beauty mark from placing my head on my mother's back. On the right side of her back she had a beauty mark that mentally rubbed off on the right side of my face. The negative association with this mole is clouded with guilt from this association with my mother and the exclusion of my sister from my mother's love.

I pushed my associations further and thought about my mother. I believed a woman (my mother) conceived by someone (me) lying on her back. My sister was born out of my act and her one eye did not focus correctly. She was, as they called it then, cross-eyed. My son had just told us that he has had a difficult time focusing and has been instructed in eye exercises to correct this. To my it, my sister and son were one person. Earlier in the day, my mind had drifted several times to my sister who lives in England. Did her daughter receive our presents? Did they get there on time?

When I grew up I always felt responsible for the travails of my sister, Judy, and cousin Bob. I was always made to feel lucky and they were struck with ill fortune. No wonder I wished them ill or worse. It was always "lucky Augie, poor Judy," as if it were my fault. (This is my interpretation, for I am sure my parents never made such causal connections.) Here I am wishing my sister ill, my son ill.

One can see the associations that led to vertigo. This malady metaphorically was a moral fall. I felt guilty about being well and healthy and guilty about my anger and jealousy towards my sick son and sick sister. I literally fell ill.

What finally triggered this drama? As I mentioned, Kazantzakis is rich in metaphor as well as family history. As I walked, I tried to recollect those last pages I read. I was reading the chapter about Nikos's father and how he paid little attention to his son, or anyone else for that matter. Only once did he compliment his son. When his son had done well at school (not disgraced his father), he threw a compliment and then drew it back. In my mind, it struck me that the father had remembered a former accusation against the son. The child (me) was guilty. Shortly thereafter in the text, Kazanzakis tells of a man daring to ask the author's father why he is so sullen. His father shot back by asking why the crow was black. The trigger was there for me. I remembered the crow as a raven, Poe's raven, black, like a beauty mark, a harbinger of death and nevermore. In the interpretation that I read into the story, the father rejected the son who was guilty and in the next breath reminded him of his beauty mark which was evidence of the son's guilt and death wish against his sister (son). The last sentence I read spoke of the paschal cake and the red egg: my sister's eye and my son's tonsils were the size of a large bird's egg.

Of course, these associations stretch my credibility with you to the limit. Remember, you wanted me to show you how this process works. This is my history and these are my associations, so these claims would not be the ones you would draw. Nevertheless, you can try to forge such associations and see if there are any similarities in the process.

Before I close this letter, let me mention one link in this story that is less certain than all the rest to me. Dr. Groddeck put into my head that children develop their own ideas about the birth process. Men may impregnate women from any orifice including the navel, and birth as well as conception may happen in that way. In my thinking about vertigo, I gave you the linkage between picking up the mole from my mother's back and making my mother pregnant. This association is very strong. So also are my feelings of guilt over my sister's eye and the feeling that my parents hold me responsible. I am jealous of my sister for she too is solicitous of my parents. The mole is evidence that I am competing for my mother over and against my sister and father. I do not need intercourse with my mother as a linkage in the story. I am not sure of this; perhaps Groddeck put the suggestions too carefully in my head. The other possibility is that I am resistant to the idea, a course I will pursue on my own. As I have described to you before in this letter, loose ends are picked up at future times, sometimes spontaneously as in the case of the mysterious mole, sometimes deliberately. At some future time, I will pick up the story where the son was left clinging on his mother's back.

Let me pursue the possibility that reading Groddeck put this idea in my head. In his writings and by example, he feels that the mother is of overwhelming import in what he finds about himself. He is indebted to Freud for the Oedipus and castration complexes. As I mentioned, he speaks of the birth myths we have as well as the mother image we create and many other structures. If we read Freud, Jung, Adler, or any of the moderns, they speak of important structures chronologically from the archetypes of Jung to the birth traumas of Rank to the oral, anal, and phallic stages of Freud to the contemporary crises of living that the moderns point out. Birth trauma for Rank is prior and more important to him than Freud's three stages of sexuality, yet a will to power supercedes these for Adler. I could go on, but these are the areas of greatest debate among analysts. What generalized structures do we find in human development? What important objects, important conflicts, important instincts, or impulses, are to be surmounted? When analysts generalize what they find in themselves and others, then they run into other analysts who find more important structures. Also, those they train or analyze look for the same structures. This is why I tell you that I remain skeptical about my birth theory in the vertigo story. It is inevitable that we find some of these structures that others have happened upon. As you can glean from my story, Oedipus lurks around the corner. I feel we must be skeptical when we uncover these heretofore known structures, maybe we find them to please Groddeck, Freud, or Sayres. Second, we must be careful not to generalize too much from them. What is important is the method of exploration. We can use what others have found, but with profound reserve. Beware the importance of the mother and Oedipus for they reign below the level of my awareness. If you find them, examine your relationship with me.

I cannot wait for your response to these letters. When we next meet, I have already steeled myself for your piercing glance at my upper lip. Surprise, for empirical evidence has it— testimony from friends and relatives—that the mole has faded. Perhaps the working of the it?

Give my respects to your mother.

Augie

———————€———————

Dear B. J.,

You are quite correct. I left many loose ends in the last two letters. I will answer your comments, but first let me tell you of happy endings. My son is out of the hospital and made a quick recovery. He left yesterday for New York. He attributes his rapid recovery to the fine Mexican restaurants in town. This provided him with a great incentive to get well enough to eat. He does not believe in my school of medicine; the decision to have his tonsils out was his and not mine. No, it does not cause me any serious problems that there is, in your words, an apostate in my house. I would be fooling myself, however, if I did not admit to myself that I would have preferred Groddeck to the knife in this instance. When you bring up children to make their own choices, there are times you wish you could call a moratorium and gather your power over them back for an instant. He is well, happy to be rid of the tonsils, and by his definition cured. I grant him that; he is a worthy opponent in discussion. You see here what I see: a frustrated father. Yes. Coerce him to Groddeck! As I return from defeat, I do so trying to learn. I am reminded again how modest we must be in what we know, how many ways there are to view the world, and how finite we are.

Enough of the prosaic father, for I have to answer your comments. You are correct in your suggestion that during the course of a day we are constructing an agenda, or, as I would put it, *ruminations,* and these resemble a dream in their fragmentary ways and wild associations. I would go further and say that if I do not unravel these ruminations at the end of the day, they would make up the better part of my dream.

As you suggest, there are many implications in ruminating. The most obvious is that what we are aware of as the most important of the day's objectives may pale in emotional intensity beside those ideas below the level of awareness. As I pointed out before, children and the elderly are most aware of these themes and, often to our annoyance, become compulsive about demands from these sources. At times, for the rest of us, the orders of the day are a facade which we can walk through to carry out the intensely important dramas. This becomes interesting because it almost reverses our notions about conscious and unconscious when we use these terms. We can carry out our daily affairs partially under hypnosis, unconsciously, while choosing from those events that impinge upon us a serious script. For example, on the day I got vertigo, my day was planned and routine. The contacts with others and the wider environment simply set the stage for an important drama: illness as a result of guilt and identification with the patient.

You make an interesting point when you say that I felt sleepy before I made the nasty statement about my son. In other words, I began to conspire with my illness before the "traumatic" statement. This allows me to comment a bit on cause and cure. For the sake of awareness, we like ideas in neat causal packages. I wish I could say that from my dramatic statement all elements were caused. A rumination may be hatched in an instant or over a lifetime; my plot had been hatched long before, as well as on that day. Acceleration of my running, subsequent thoughts about dizziness and fatigue, and my sick son—one I should have had sympathy for—set up a rumination that for me is a classic. I had appealed to my son to understand illness as I do, he had rejected me, and I was annoyed. My wife had shown great sympathy for my son. In my mind it was lucky Augie and poor son (Judy, Bob) all over again, a plot hatched years before. Even before the day began, I was disposed to search for a creative solution. I searched out all the elements for the rest of the day. Humdrum events of the day help one make up the rumination; they fill in the details, confirm one's suspicions, suggest new approaches— all to play variations on a theme.

These are the dynamics of creative ruminations, but they do not answer your key questions: when did the vertigo go away and why? In answer to the first, it obviously went away when I was walking. Many of the ends and threads of the rumination came out during the walk. All of them were not necessary for the alleviation of symptoms. The statement I had made about my son hit me as critical as I brought it to awareness. I had said

it with dramatic flair and it was surrounded by an aura of un-
reality. Although it was only one element in the rumination,
certainly neither the first nor the the last, it was the action which
made the rumination of consequence.

The answer to the question, Why? is that my vertigo disappeared when I dealt with my statement to my son. As you know,
psychoanalysts have felt for a long time now that awareness is
no longer a guarantee of a cure. To this I heartily agree. (You
will see in my work this question has come to interest me greatly.) Even a full picture of the underlying dynamics does not
necessarily bring change. What I would like to say to bring a
magic cure is: "Look at the fable I have created. As an adult I
have created or re-created a situation that recurred in my
childhood. Now I am an adult and I realize my son is my son;
my wife, my wife; my father is in Florida and doesn't even know
my son is having his tonsils out and, of course, doesn't have any
idea or could care less what I said to my wife."

What I find, however, is that I often have to act to remedy
the situation. Sometimes the symptoms disappear if I convince
myself that I will in time absolutely follow a course of action
I prescribe. At other times, and I will give you an example, I
have to actually do the action before change occurs. This time
I was lucky, because when the prescription occurred to me on
the walk and I convinced myself I would act on it, the symptoms disappeared. Most often the prescription calls for communication with a specific person or persons. In this case, I was
going to repeat to my wife the statement I made about my son.
Then I would tell her how it was not a reflection on him, but
a reflection on me. It occurs to me now that it allows me to say,
"Judy's all right, it's Augie's fault," which is far less difficult on
me than what the statement implied to me in the first place,
"Judy's a loser and Augie's OK." Once I was certain I would
make this confession, the symptoms disappeared.

Often, as I said, I have to take the action before the symptom or symptoms disappear. This time I was lucky, but I can
relate another time when I was not so lucky. I was teaching a
summer institute with several others, and I came up with a
screaming headache while watching *Porky's,* a movie I had
rented to play on the VCR. My wife was in New York visiting

her relatives. My crime was multiple: I was watching TV without permission—a tacky movie as well—and by watching the movie, I was not attending the party given by the person who organized the institute. I realized the headache would go away once I apologized for not attending the party. The headache was severe and even the proposed solution did not alter the pain in any way. The next day, I saw the hostess and made a full confession. (She was aware of Groddeck.) I apologized for not attending the party and told her why I was apologizing. Within thirty minutes my headache, still as severe as it had been the prior night, disappeared.

I have asked myself why it did not disappear when I made plans to apologize. Perhaps I was not convinced I would actively seek her out and apologize the next day. As I was writing this section to you, it occurred to me that I might not have planned to tell her the whole story. If I knew that I would not make a full confession, then the headache would remain. The old mind-cure expert Dale Carnegie told us to take action even if we did not believe in it and eventually we would convince ourselves. We can render no such tricks on the it.

If I am convinced that certain steps are inevitable, then I can alleviate symptoms immediately. Otherwise, the cure must await the action.

I have finished my saga of vertigo and I wait for your reply.

Your friend,

Augie

Letters to Mom

Dear Mom,

All through the years you have shown great concern that perhaps you did not bring up my sister and me correctly. This has caused you much grief. I intend to show that you need not have worried and certainly you should no longer worry. Even though you abdicated your authority to Dr. Spock, Sigmund Freud, and other childrearing luminaries of the day, their advice was heeded with goodwill. When the authority was your own, you proceeded to do what you thought best for us. Judy and I, as much as I can presume to speak for her, must each take the responsibility for our own life and existence.

Perhaps I can show you how much of your guilt was unnecessary if I can explain to you how you suffered much over what was not your own fault. Of course, I am referring to my "stomach problems." Ever since I was a child I can remember having difficulties. I even hid the worst from you. When I was in high school, I had diarrhea and always thought of myself as a profile in courage. Those basketball trips I made were extraordinarily difficult because I had to "hold it in" until we got to the opponent's gym. Once there, I even worried about having to leave the game and go to the bathroom. One time when I was going to track practice, I failed to hold it in and, in total shame, ran home without telling anyone why. I threw my pants and undergarments in the garbage and held on to my secret.

You did your best for me in those days. I can remember you and Grandma traveling a half hour each way to get me acidophilus milk to cure my stomach. If the taste did not cure me, nothing would. You took me to specialists who gave me bluish medicine, pills, and other medications to help me. This is on top of the over-the-counter remedies of Kaopectate and Pepto Bismol. I must have consumed gallons of the chalky liquid and the sweet pink fluid that blackened the tongue. Nothing seemed to work for long, but none of it was your fault. You did not want for trying.

I did my best to hide the pain from you, but I am sure you had to think about my problem when you saw the pink pockets of my pants where the Pepto Bismol tablets had crumbled. Those tablets were a great innovation for me, though probably a cause of annoyance and concern for you. I could pop one of those tablets every time I felt cramps coming on. This was a convenience that bottles would never allow. As a teenager, I could never carry a flask of Kaopectate or Pepto Bismol around. (Curious were the objects of such great concern to me.) I remember when our family physician said that it was probably in my mind and I ought to go to a psychiatrist. I bristled at the thought. Another called it a problem of nerves. If there was anything a teenager of that time could not abide, it was to be considered nervous, not cool. I was the one admired for having ice water in my veins when I played sports. Certainly I was not nervous. I know that you felt these "nerves" theories had the most credence. You told me in many ways at different times that you pushed me too hard to play sports and I was put in too many pressure situations. I refused to pay any heed to any hypothesis that hit at my esteem or sanity.

As I look back, you were both right and wrong. You and the doctors were correct that my life and circumstances did play a great role in my illness. But I was not disposed at that time to accept that view. I was better able to accept outside forces, or those beyond my control, as the cause of my problem. I preferred to believe that I was missing an essential enzyme, harbored intestinal bacteria, had an allergy, or was overly prone to the twenty-four-hour virus. It's true. I held these hypotheses at different times in my life. You were correct in suspecting an internal cause. I know you suspect as much in yourself, but have never taken any action on that basis. Instead, you have armed yourself to treat yourself and others with an arsenal of pills. Sometimes you were able to alleviate symptoms, and I was grateful in college for the Lomotil I got from you to treat my stomach problems. Through college and until recent years I denied having any stomach problems, yet I carried around those precious little white pills as the ultimate stopper. If all else failed (Pepto Bismol tablets in more plentiful supply were used first), I would go to the little white pill. You were doubly correct: the cause may be internal and symptoms may be greatly relieved by medication.

Where you were wrong and caused yourself needless grief was in your assumption that you knew the cause of my discomfort—stress—and that you caused it. You felt that those pressures to play and compete caused my discomfort. The answer I continued to give you was correct. If games were tight or exams were upcoming, my stomach ceased to be a problem. In the former case, I could not think about my stomach, and in the latter, my appetite decreased drastically. I tried in other situations to divert attention from my stomach and also tried to eat less, but neither was a permanent cure. Nonetheless, I was correct in indicating (as I will show you further on) that pressure situations did not aggravate my stomach. All the guilt you suffered from thinking this was not necessary. In those early years, you did an excellent job in trying to help me solve my stomach problems. You took me to the best specialists, and treatment went from pills to bluish fluids to barium enemas. These remedies could scarcely do more than temporarily alleviate symptoms. My guess is that the guilt you felt, and probably still feel, must come from believing you were part of the cause and not because you stopped short of finding a cure.

I point all of this out to show you the difficulties of blaming yourself for the ills of others. I have come to realize that each individual is, with training, best able to explain sources of his or her own behavior. But a parent may have to guide the child who is helpless to deal with his or her problems. If the child is not aware of the source of the problem, and does not communicate, the parents are left only with poor guesses. Your theory was correct: the cause was internal. This brilliant insight caused you only grief for you thought you knew the specific cause. Here was the basis of error and grief.

Even if you had no such feelings of guilt over being the cause, I know the frustrations of being a parent and being able to do nothing about suffering. Perhaps it gets back again to the idea of cause when we assume that through evolution or our behavior we brought on the condition. The victim, in this case the child, may place the blame on the outside source, the parent. The child plays on the parent's guilt and looks to obtain sympathy. No, I do not blame myself either. It is only now that I am aware of these principles.

Why do we have difficulty guessing the cause of ills of others? More on that later. Now it remains to tell you of my own futile attempts at trying to solve the mysteries of my illness. When I went to work in New York at Price Waterhouse, I had to take the subway from Brooklyn. This was a time of terror for me because my stomach was so bad in the morning. The crowds were massive, and often the trains were so packed that I had to let several of them go by so that I could squeeze on. I remember getting on the train and having fear of being trapped in the middle of the car by hordes of people and not being able to get off in time. I knew where every toilet was on the BMT line from Flatbush Avenue to Whitehall Street. Many times I made use of them; at all times I was acutely aware of my options. By the time I got to work I felt the heroic surge of one who held off the enemy, the absurdity of my conquest, and the exhaustion from my efforts. It was not even difficult to practice accounting, a job I was unsuited for, after such heroic exertion. When I went back to study at the university, I was afraid that if I got out and taught I would never be able to make it for fifty minutes in front of a class. Many times while I was attending a class, it would be a *cliffhanger* to stay until the end of the period.

I did not pick up on the selectivity of my illness towards situation and place. As you know, I began seeing the demons in foods and was treated for food allergies. As with other cures, I had some successes. Now I have dealt with the cause interna and need to complete that story. This will have to await my next letter. In the meantime, I am aware of your skepticism, for I have always tried to semi-hide the "stomach problems" from you. As you see, now I am trying to be as candid as I can.

As I look back on all these experiences, what becomes obvious is that with a toilet readily nearby and accessible, my problems were less than when I was isolated and feared an accident. In *Portnoy's Complaint,* I had read Philip Roth's description of the protagonist's living in fear that his mother would find a "wisp of shit" in his underpants he left for washing. We have great fear of such things in our society. If that had been my only fear.

Love,

Augie

Dear Mom,

In your letter you seemed pleased that I have found a solution to my stomach problems. I do sense a skepticism in the tone of your letter, and that is acceptable to me. No longer do I feel that we can convince others of our views. All I can do is state my position with clarity and candor. Much more serious is your comment that I "tormented" you with half of the story and that you cannot wait for my conclusion. I reread my letter to you and feel that your choice of words was appropriate. You describe a pattern that I have followed all my life and have found in others. I snap you to attention with some dramatic happening, looking for sympathy and interest, and then in my own time and fashion, I dramatically release you from fear. On the surface, your torment is my withholding a promising conclusion, but there is much more to this presentation of *cliffhangers*. In the letter I make it known to you that my problems were worse than you suspected, and I startled you with the accident on the track and with the language I cited from the Philip Roth book. The easy way out would be to say that I merely wanted to remind you of my stomach problem or to clarify it for myself, but these are only rationalizations. You have always viewed my stomach problems as serious, and I have pre-thought this example dozens of times in my mind. I was taking you on a dramatic ride, an adventure, one that solidifies our destinies.

I have a student who is very mild mannered and respectful to his parents. Oddly enough, he is an avid rock climber and has hurt himself seriously in climbing. After some discussion, he admits that he is playing to his mother, even if she is five hundred miles away. Give me a daredevil and behind him I will find someone who is preparing cliffhangers for his mother. My old friend Groddeck understood this all too well in his analysis of Ibsen's *Peer Gynt*. Peer Gynt comes home and tells his mother about holding on to the antlers of a deer on a thin edge of a precipice of a mountain. His mother is captivated and enthralled by Peer's story until she realizes he is lying. Cliffhangers are for our mothers, and we play them out all of our lives hoping that, even if not present, our mothers will hear of our exploits. We may risk illness or injury to captivate our mothers. Sometimes we do fall off the precipice into a well of sympathy and concern. In no way are mothers responsible for these dramatic shows, but they do play a role in our illnesses. Once I have understood who my audience is, I can better modulate my performance. Do not feel guilty about playing a part in this dynamic. We fall, and are not pushed, off the precipice.

You are probably saying again that by giving you the logic of cliffhangers I am accentuating the cliffhanger. Why not save this analysis for the denouement? I could have, but the impulse to create cliffhangers is too great. With great difficulty, in order to cause no further torment, I will proceed from the graphic descriptions of my stomach problems to the solution.

When I left to teach in England for those five months, I still had stomach problems. I was no longer willing to put up with them. My self-analysis began on my one-hour jogs through Regent's Park. The wonderful setting, the quiet early hours, and the routine of two lazy loops around the park allowed me to free associate. Each day I would push a bit closer to the root of the problem. I went back to the time of the "accident" and told myself that many worse events could happen to a person. I imagined myself having such an "accident" in every conceivable place and found no event that I could not handle. The fear involved in searching for a deeper solution began to lessen and associations were more forthcoming.

Some of the fits and starts I made in my search have faded from my memory, but after several weeks, from my childhood flashed a picture of cousin Bob seated on the toilet and my seeing something purple. I could make out concern on everyone's face at Bob's plight, and yet I did not know why. Some weeks later, as I continued self-analysis, it popped into my head that I had not been seeing testicles. (All my reading of Freud convinced me that I should have found them—my fault, not Freud's.) Actually, I had seen Bob's colon partially out of his body.

Aha! Now you know why I asked you about that event. You confirmed my recollection and said that Bob had a distended colon. You were amazed that I could remember something that had happened so long ago. Now we get at the crux of my stomach problems. No one was aware of the presence of the older cousin, for the concern was with the younger, as the doctor tried to tease the colon back in place. Curiosity got the better of the child that I was, and I put my own creative meaning to the story. Before you blame yourself for my being present at the event that happened so long ago, let me point out that as a youngster I saw dogs killed, men die, women screaming in pain, children beaten, and many other childhood horrors. Children have shocking experiences; they cannot be protected from such occurrences. I was the one who put the particular interpretation on this event. My own creativity was the cause of my stomach affliction. Mothers and fathers cannot protect their children from every possibility of trauma in their lives. A child may steal a brownie from the kitchen and a sister be blamed for the theft. The guilty one, silent, may suffer from the event for the rest of his life, while the other parties to the incident have long since forgotten it. Goodness knows you tried to protect us, but our its are too creative and life offers too many chances to ever protect anyone completely. There is no one to blame here.

Let me explain for a moment why Bob's travail became so important in my life. I interpreted his problem to mean that we all have plugs in our colon and we could lose them. I witnessed all the horror and consternation that occurs when it happens. Although the event tended to symbolize different things as I began to learn of anatomy, the metaphor of the plug was always to concern me. In those early years, I was not sure what shape or form it was. For most of my life, the plug was a well-formed bowel movement. If I had any movement that was loose, I assumed there was no more plug and I was in trouble. Before I went anywhere I would go and go, hoping to empty the contents of my system so all would not leak out.

If I were to be going someplace where I would not have access to a toilet, I would always test to see if a plug existed. The problem was that it was a nontestable proposition: if I went and a firm plug came out, what guarantees that another plug existed? I would listen to my system and fear that disaster was not far away. I know how foolish this sounds, but such are the tricks of the it.

My rehabilitation came when I threw out the metaphor of the plug. Once I replaced this false imagery with an accurate picture of the way the system worked and the realization that I had created my own fears, my problem went away. I still have to remind myself of the metaphor, and scars of the experience remain, but I am well. No longer is any trip to a movie or play, vacation, or stint in front of a classroom an adventure in the way it was before. If you want proof that I am well, observe that my reluctance to venture forth has vanished.

A critical test I worked for myself was in Athens when we were traveling the Continent. I agreed to go on a bus to Delphi, three and one-half hours from Athens. The driver did not speak English, because this was not a tourist bus. I did not know if the driver was going to stop at all. He did stop once. I told myself the worst that could happen and got on the bus. There was no looking for the plug, no panic that my stomach was about to explode. The journey there and back was uneventful. I still remember my experience whenever such a situation occurs. But there is no more panic, just reminders that I am well, there are no plugs, and we create our own discomfort.

I obviously shortened the story for there is more to my relationship with Bob, many intermediate steps to that traumatic scene, and the dead ends along the way. Sometime I will fill you in on the details. Now they would obscure what I am trying to explain. You may rest for I am well. My adventures over the years probably took some glow off your life. I cannot blame myself, for cliffhangers were below my level of awareness. Now I can no longer play the same game. If we want to show how uncertain blame is, from a family perspective, my stomach problems might have deflected your attention from some other situation where you felt even less efficacious and more frustrated.

We cannot judge ourselves or others in these matters. Often trivial events, ones that other people handle routinely, can cause us trouble in later life. Our interpretations are unique. My particular relationship to my cousin, a particular age when I was theorizing about bowel function, seeing the ineffectualness of adults were all interwoven into an explanation that should not make us to feel guilty, but to laugh. How creative to dream up a plug!

In a letter to a mother from a son, I can try to allay anxieties. I am aware, however, that cliffhangers are an established pattern, and I may have set some cliffhangers even as I was trying to allay your fears—a common trick. Judge not for I do not do so on purpose.

To care and good intentions.

Augie

PS. To show how deep these cliffhangers go, I will tell you in English the only full sentence of Russian I remember from the hundreds I once knew: "I slipped and fell and almost broke my foot."

Dear Mom,

    I see from your letter that you continue to worry about me. These feelings are all part of the cliffhangers we have played out over the years. Your grandson Martin plays them with his mother. You know the letters of disaster that children send home from camp. I am sure I sent a few. Martin sent home a letter which described his activities in glowing terms. Coincidentally, Jimmy Cohen fell off the top of a double-decker bed and had to be sent home. Not a word about where Martin sleeps. We will worry for Martin's safety and that is his message. I wish we could communicate directly sometimes. He should say to his mother, "Assure me that you won't forget me while I am at camp." Or as I should say to you, "Don't forget me. I am as interesting and as much fun as I was at the age of twelve."

    Separations and reunions are dangerous times for people. My nephew Cal went to camp and felt a bit abandoned by his parents, who are separated. Predictably he got sick, but attention was not forthcoming. His letters home pleaded indirectly for attention, but when his parents called the camp, they were assured that he was well cared for. A few weeks went by and he was still ill. The mother and then the father visited—Cal's mission accomplished. The child had lost considerable weight and this had gone unnoticed by the camp. His usual protest at home is to eat in a picky fashion. It is a means of power over his family. The trick did not work at camp; they ignored his picky habits. The payoff for him was when his parents came on the emergency visit. Within a day or two he was well.

    I know what you are going to say. How can I know the dynamics long distance? Yet, I am hesitant to give you examples from my own life, for you will be forced to play cliffhangers again. Here is another example, one closer to home. I asked Martin if he understood how illnesses work. He said that he gets sick infrequently. I asked when the last time was that he was sick, and he said last May. Before he was supposed to go to Boys' State, he got a severe sore throat. His analysis was as follows: he was supposed to finish school, participate in Boys' State for a week, and go off to the camp the day after his return. At the time, he was agitated, and how he protested going to Boys' State! The privilege is bestowed upon the students and is supposed to be looked upon as an honor. For a teen, it is difficult to turn down the honor due to pressure from his friends and, perhaps in his mind, fear of disappointing his parents. He kept reflecting how he had nothing to say to these people; he was not interested in politics. A sore throat was a creative solution. He got out of going to Boys' State, recovered quickly, and had several days to rest before heading off to be a counselor at camp. All this was done to an orchestrated symphony of sympathy. The literature on stress will reinforce my point that vacations, departures, and reunions are deleterious to one's health.

Now I can tell you what is utmost on my mind, although I have no ultimate hopes of persuading you. I give you the examples of my own illnesses and those of others to show you how the it weaves it's merry tales. Ultimately, I am hoping that you will turn to analyzing yourself. I am most concerned when you decide to go on a trip about which you have ambivalent feelings. You do not like to admit to housing such feelings, but we all have them. When I visit you, there is for me the joy of anticipating the visit plus the trepidation of the ill feelings that may unfold, the difficulties in doing what the group wants, and many other feelings of concern both above and below awareness. To avoid accident or illness, it is necessary to explore such feelings fully, otherwise, some accident or illness will befall you! Need I remind you that you cut the tendon in your thumb just before you went overseas to visit Judy? The next year you planned to go to Greece with Carole and me but got so sick to your stomach that you had to cancel. Then you went to Greece later and on your own route.

Let me speak of that because I may have some insight. In a moment of candor, you admitted that the whole package of figs that you ate probably contributed to your troubles. We all laughed when I said a package that large would give an elephant a bellyache. Remember that before we went we changed our plans several times and you were really agitated about many aspects of the plan. The stomachache was a creative solution. You went off later on your own at your own time, and we were not angry at you for the change of plans, but sympathetic.

Why am I telling you this? As you know, we all feel the obligation (out of guilt or altruism—I will not go into this now) of helping others. I no longer see accidents or illness as twists of fate, irony, and absurdity. Today, I cannot laugh at the fig incident, for it was no mistake. On some level it was deliberate on your part. So you see, I can no longer let such an incident slide by when I see you in danger.

Also, I know that you are aware of the mechanism of which I speak. You were aware that the cause was internal when I was ill. All those years you insisted it was nerves or stress. Very often, however, we are giving advice not to others, but to ourselves. You were telling yourself that you were the cause of your own ills. When I tell you all of this about the dangers of travel and reunion, I am also warning myself. Now I look at all advice as dual; I am advising others, but primarily myself. For example, as my children were growing up, I gave them very little sympathy when they were ill. My daughter was bitter over this for a long while. I felt that they would get better quicker if they got no sympathy. I was really talking about myself, because I thrived on your sympathy when I was ill. You lavished it on me. My fear was when grandma would come as arbiter to check on my swollen glands, to see if my throat was red or my nose was stuffed. This was not what I wanted. I thrived on *your* sympathy. It made the illness worth it.

If you accept the cause interna, the next step is much more difficult. Why would you give yourself a stomachache to get out of going on the trip? It meant suffering the pain of the illness as well as the inconvenience of making new reservations when you and Dad went later. This solution does not hold up to rational analysis. I agree, but the it does not weigh consequences in that manner. You were agitated about going on the trip and you successfully avoided going. Although one pain not need match another, below the level of awareness the trip was painful.

Notice that I have avoided giving you a specific explanation for your unhappiness. This is the kind of analysis one must do for oneself. If I were to guess—and it is always tempting—I would probably be no closer to an explanation than you were when you felt that I got stomach problems when I went into competitive situations. Our guesses for others, as I suggest, are often for ourselves. In recent years you have told me how difficult it is for you to compete in golf tournaments and other athletic events. More likely this problem of nerves in competitive situations was your problem and not mine. But then, this is only my guess.

You will have to do the analysis yourself, without any help. I would give my advice to you as I do to others if you would take it in the proper spirit. That would be for you to say, "You are dead wrong, Augie, but. . . ." Still, I am better off restraining myself. If I collected all the advice I have given over the years, I would have written my autobiography.

I have no doubt that you will see the cause interna in others; believe it for yourself. However, I still see a reluctance on your part to make a self-analysis. This means coming to grips with negative feelings which you are loathe to admit you may have about people. I would accept Will Rogers's saying that he never met a man he did not like, if he also said he never met a man he liked.

I hope you enjoy your trip and make it in health and safety.

Love,

Augie

PS. Please use the letter to see if your feelings towards me are ambiguous—as well they should be. I love you and I am angry with you for I know you will reject much of what I say. As a discipline, and after much practice, I judge not.

Letters to B. J.

Dear B. J.,

I am glad to know you are pleased with my letters. You are correct that in the past I wrote less frequently. Your speculations on my motives are intriguing when you guessed that my newer friends were more vital to me, that perhaps we had grown apart over the years, or even that I was angry with you over something you said. I was particularly interested in your speculations because I am so curious about what passes between people. My life is full of such speculations about human relations. What I have come to suspect is that our guesses about others reveal more about ourselves. See if what you surmised about our correspondence is really an expression of your own feelings.

To illustrate what I mean, I will draw an example from my own experience. Some time ago I picked up my good friend Michael at the airport. He was to be in town for two days to give a talk. Each of four of us from campus was at the airport to pick up a friend who was to speak at this four-day conference. When the airplane came in, I grabbed Mike, ignored my local colleagues and their guests, and rushed him out of there. One of these local colleagues was with his guest, and as Mike and I were leaving, I made eye contact with my colleague.

On the way back to town from the airport, Mike and I were already engaged in talk about Groddeck, finitude, and candor, concerns that we have in common. Finally, I told him what was weighing on my mind. I had snubbed this friend at the airport, and when our eyes met, he showed his anger and disapproval at my snub. Mike's response, the correct one, was that I probably misread the situation. We often speak past one another. Nonetheless, the incident continued to bother me, and I was all too aware of this rumination that was spoiling the rest of my day.

My inclination is to speak directly to someone to straighten out such situations. When I saw this friend that I had snubbed at the airport, I readied myself to make an apology. It was to be a milder variant of "Sorry, I can see you any time, and I want to spend as much time as I can with Mike." I was withdrawn into my rumination and fashioning my apology when this campus friend spoke first, "Sorry, Augie, I saw you at the airport, but didn't stop for introductions. We were in a hurry to get out of the airport and get back to town." Mike was correct; I had obviously misread this friend's motives. He was not angry with me but was feeling guilty because he had pulled the same stunt I had.

We so often misread other people and see our motives in them or, as in the case above, make them coconspirators to the games we are playing in our own heads. This is a very long way of saying that those were not my motives for being a poor correspondent in the past. Perhaps you felt your friends had become more vital to you than old Augie. Or you were feeling guilty because we had grown apart. Possibly you were angry with me. All these feelings may be wrapped up in a rumination of your own. I would be foolish to guess as to a final answer. What I am trying to do is to show you how we think. We guess motives and advice ends up on the ash heap. If we are to make anything of our advice or guesses, we should use them to understand ourselves. All of this is a prelude to explaining why I have been such a poor correspondent. Do not judge yourself to be at fault. I will show you why my missives were few and far between. My parsimony as a correspondent does tend to seem puzzling since I write for a living.

What I am going to tell you is that part of the reason that I have not written often is that I was cursed. This is something that you could have no awareness of. Before you deliver me to Salem to be exorcized, let me explain what the dynamics of the situation are. The term *curse,* as you will see, is my own and bears no mystical connotations.

If you notice, I say "part of the reason," because the problem of not writing is a complex one and involves more than the curse. If you read my article on writing, you will complete the picture. I must set up for you the circumstances that occurred when the curse was pronounced. When we were together years ago, I spoke very little of my future plans. I was to become, like my father, an accountant. Ruminations had already set in and I had hoped to do something else with my life. I majored in economics in college and took plenty of accounting courses. The initial choice of schools reflected my ambivalence. I chose a school where you could not major in accounting, but you could take some courses in it. What a hedge, when there were many schools accessible to me that offered full accounting degrees. This was one of those choices that hover on the brink of aware-ness to break in only at times. After a year and a half in the army, I went to work at Price Waterhouse. My best friend there was Bob Newhart, the comedian, someone I had never met. He had escaped from accounting to an entirely different career. After working there for a year, I applied for graduate school and was accepted.

The inevitable was that I had to tell my father that I was leaving accounting to go into the teaching profession. In my mind, this meant a great disappointment for him. At Price Waterhouse I was gaining the experience to take over his firm. He took the news calmly enough. Like a good father, he began to inquire to see if I had thought this adventure through. On the one hand, I had little money, no assistantship to begin with, and a wife and small child to support; on the other, I had the promise of a lucrative career in accounting, either with his firm or Price Waterhouse. You can imagine how badly I answered his questions. Simmel's very definition of an adventure, which I had no knowledge of at the time, is facing a situation with no ready answers. I was not prepared to say to my father that I had no answers and that the uncertainty was the very adventure of it all, the excitement as well. So, I tried as best I could to show in balance-sheet fashion that this adventure really was not an adventure at all.

I had made up my mind to go back to school, and I was not going to be bothered by his questions or by what would seem to him ridiculous answers. We began to discuss what it meant to be a college teacher. He told me that I would not make much money and that it was not a competitive field (it may, however, be an easy life), and he offered other descriptive ideas—some positive, some negative—about college teaching. My recollec-tion of this part of the conversation is sketchy, but I am willing to bet those descriptions were more of what I thought he would say rather than what he actually said.

None of the discussion was conducted like an inquisition. We had a concerned father who was asking the questions he should have asked in such a situation. My father, as you know, is mild mannered and I have never (childhood idealization?) seen him lose his temper. (Another digression—it is interesting that we lose our temper [temperance] and it is not externally taken away). Back to the story. Despite my father's reasonable approach, I felt like it was an interrogation of the guilty. I had decided to abandon his profession thereby demeaning his work and leaving him without an heir. (No pun intended. I know he is bald.) Besides, I had given him no advance warning that I would leave accounting and go back to school.

I can see as I re-read this letter that I have made many digressions (this paragraph is another one) as I come to the curse. After I finish with the curse, I will come back to the digressions, for they are interesting in their own right. Classic psychoanalysts might say that I am meeting resistance, but we may look at it in another way. As we close in on a critical event in life, our associations become richer and more productive. For now I will return to the curse and show you later how productive these digressions are.

I was feeling guilty and defensive because I was betraying my father. As he asked me about the teaching profession and alternately told me what to expect, I felt anxiety mount. At one point—for me it was the final point for I remember no other one—he asked, "HOW DO YOU EXPECT TO SUCCEED IF YOU HATE TO WRITE?" Here was the curse.

There are many comments I need to make on the idea of a curse. I have developed the concept of the curse by listening to others. We all have curses cast upon us; more importantly, we are all willing to receive them. After finding them almost universally in others, I found this one in my possession. Most often we gain access to our own life when we listen to others. Our attention wanders and unselfconsciously we begin to free associate. Groddeck's writings are most suggestive to me in this way. This curse came to me quickly.

The one who delivers the curse may or may not do so with malice or knowledge of the consequences it may have for the other person. My father was asking very sensible questions about my future plans. I suspect he does not even remember our conversation or, especially, making that remark. He would be appalled, and unnecessarily so, as you shall see, if he knew what difficulties this curse caused me.

As you would suspect from my stoic philosophy, the key is the way the person receives the message. We throw out millions of messages to other people; many are even deliberately thrown out as curses or as the counter, *blessings*. You are good, kind, generous, thoughtful, considerate—therefore, you will be these things in the future as well. You cannot spell, are rotten, spoiled, childish, selfish—carry this baggage into the future. The key is how we receive these messages. Do not judge the sender. In my case, I was feeling terribly guilty about leaving the accounting profession. My father hit on the one point where I had the most doubt. I did not like to write. I could thereafter enjoy all other aspects of the academic world except for the writing. There seems to be a principle of economy here. A curse allows us to focus all of our guilt toward one object. Instead of feeling a vague malaise about everything in my chosen profession, my father doomed me to throw all my guilt and energies into the prospect of writing. Of course, the curse confirmed my darkest suspicion: I did not like to write.

One of the major consequences of a curse is to try to overcome it. My ostensive reality is the classroom, the family, the daily routine. The actual time I spend writing, as it is for most academics, is not that time consuming. Yet, as I look back on my years in academia, my ruminations about writing were one of the central concerns of my life. When I am reading, writing, or biking, I am not putting off shaving, planning whether to use an electric razor or my disposable, deciding to shave from chin up or sideburns down. Yet, when I shave, jog, bike, teach, or cook dinner, I am always ruminating about writing, much of the time mired in guilt. Even though I have had no real awareness of the curse, I have done my best to try to overcome it.

Of course, academia places fear in the hearts of its foot soldiers, and the cry "publish or perish" is heard everywhere. I could have chosen to ignore most of this and to teach in a small private college. Given the route I took, I could have chosen to ignore the call to publish in all the years that have passed since I got tenure. The curse magnified the doctrine of publish or perish for me. Every effort to write was an attempt to overcome the curse: the thesis, books, articles, memos, and, of course, letters to you. Every word, every sentence was to overcome the curse that I hate to write.

Obviously, a curse can have outside reinforcement as my particular one has had. Also, we pick an utterance up as a curse because we may already have perceived it as a weakness. I did not particularly like to write. More on this curse and others in my next letter. Comments on my digressions will also have to wait.

The prompt arrival of my next letter will be some evidence to you that the curse has been lifted.

Augie

Dear B. J.,

As I promised, I am writing to you promptly. You are correct that my example seemed incomplete, and you wonder what I mean by blessings. I promised you that I would explain some of the digressions I made as I approached the story of my curse.

The first digression came when I stated my father was "mild mannered and I have never (childhood idealization?) seen him lose his temper." He never outwardly raged, but as with everyone, there were moments of annoyance. If someone does not outwardly lose his temper, you look for signs that he is angry. In many ways, we fear the wrath of those who rarely or never lose their temper more than those who show us their anger and expose their power resources. Talcott Parsons describes the concept of gold bullion as a resource backing up the financial system. No wonder Parsons's gold bullion and potential force are such interesting concepts for me. The idea of secret consciousness in *Character* also has, for me, its strength in that it describes the father's secret resources.

As I approached an explanation of my curse and recalled the conversation with my father, I began to make associations that showed I feared his ever possible but never forthcoming rage. My mind flashed back to the basement of the apartment house I lived in as a child. My father was angry because I had done something wrong, and he blocked my exit from the basement. Although he had never laid a hand on me, I felt he, with his secret consciousness and gold bullion of force saved up, would really hit me this time. The confrontation with my father over career choice conjured up unforeseeable consequences. It was to my great relief at the time that he pronounced the curse, for it allowed me to focus attention on this punishment. The diversion I made in my last letter when approaching the curse was not what is classically called resistance but an attempt on my part to fully describe the situation.

When I made the pun about hair-heir, I was resurrecting the one place as a child I was permitted to criticize my father, to bring him down from perfection. Conversations about his lack of hair hurt his feelings (from my perspective); he would seem to get annoyed but not lose his temper. These were attempts on my part to minimize the influence his views would have on me. If I could destroy his credibility, then I would be free to act as my own agent. This disgression again tells you something of my state of mind at the time I spoke to him about leaving accounting. I tried to minimize, as recently as my last letter and with little success, the impact of what he was going to say to me.

When we approach a topic of highly emotional content, we may increase the number of parapraxes (slips of the tongue), digressions, and clarifications. (I prefer to look at these digressions as attempting to fully clarify the situation for myself.) The incident is so rife with association that our mind or pen travels in many directions. The sociologist George Simmel often looks at one concept in social life—for instance, money in *The Philosophy of Money*—to help exhaust the meaning in life. One concept explored from all angles may tell more about society than thousands of disparate descriptions. On the level of the individual, Simmel's method abides. One incident, in this case the curse, can reveal a tremendous amount about my life and awareness. The trick is, as Freud suggests with free association, not to look at any utterance as irrelevant, insignificant, or unrelated.

Perhaps at another time I will show you where all these associations take me. For now, I will continue to elaborate around the curse to show you its dynamics. Just bear in mind that this is a boundary I put on the letter and not on my associations. If I continued on all the associations here, you would get to know more of my life and awareness than you might want.

The curse was the pulling together of a number of ideas. Like many brought up in this culture, I was not eager to write. I remember my teacher punishing every member of the class when I was in an early grade. We were told to write a composition as punishment. The teacher looked like my father's mother, hence my father, to me. In high school, I was not placed in the honors English class. Several of us rebelled and brought our resentment to the attention of the teachers. These early experiences seemed to anticipate the curse. More likely, the curse summarized and economically stated my feelings about writing—my fears, insecurities, and resentments.

After I was cursed, you saw what a strain all of these experiences were on me. My ruminations were often on this problem. In a paper entitled "Why I Hate to Write," I suggested that speaking was easy because our speech is forgotten once uttered. If a tape recorder is running, then we tend to become careful about what we say and much more inhibited in our expression. I went on to state that on paper we can look at ourselves and judge ourselves as to whether we are good or bad as writers and as persons.

In my article, I may have been describing a universal difficulty with writing, but I realize it had for me a definite historical meaning. My father would ultimately judge whether I could write well or not. He had cursed me and I fought against his curse. Everything I wrote I prejudged, knowing that ultimately it would have to be approved by my father. Now you can see why, before I understood the curse, I had given the job of editing my work to my father. On some level I understood that all my writing had to undergo his scrutiny. To facilitate this I gave him my work to read. My anxiety was lessened to know when and where he would judge. Today I am free to choose an editor and still choose my father, for he does an excellent job. The anxiety is no longer there, however.

Using Simmel's principle of uncovering all through full exploration of one incident or concept, what I call a *nexus,* let me illustrate a blessing through the same incident. My father would always tell me to take a career/job that I would enjoy. "Do a job you enjoy." This was the blessing and it was backed up by several family legends. My father's mother had told each of her sons what profession he would pursue—one was to be a lawyer, one was to support the others through school, and my father was to be an accountant. Here is an instance of a *blessing/ curse* a generation back. The injunctions were so strong that all landed in the professions dictated by the mother. One of the brothers strayed but returned in later life to the profession chosen for him.

Whether something is a blessing or a curse depends on the valuation we put on it after we discover its existence. I may judge my father's brothers successful, but each of them must decide whether he is blessed or cursed. My father repeatedly told me that he would have chosen to be an architect if he had it to choose all over again. Architecture was more creative to him than accounting and remained an unfulfilled dream. Yet my father is successful as an accountant. In retirement now, he has chosen to continue doing accounting. My father was blessed/cursed and told to be an accountant. He always told me to do something I enjoyed. Rarely, however, are blessings/curses unambiguous. He prospered as an accountant in the face of his own advice to me.

Now that I have told you about this blessing you can see full well why I left accounting. The only surprise might be why I tried accounting at all. I was frightened of my father; there was the idea of gold bullion, the fear of his unexpressed wrath. But why should I fear leaving accounting when my father is telling me to do what I enjoy? Clearly, the message was mixed for me, because my father continued to work as an accountant. In a reverie about this situation, it occurred that my father was sincere all those years when he asked me, "Why did you go into accounting? Did you think I wanted it for you? I really wanted to be an architect!"

Correct! My father was sincere. My mother wanted me to be an accountant for she thought it would please my father. (This is my interpretation of what happened.) My mother thought this would please my father, to perpetuate his name, to forge closer ties between a very busy father and his son. I followed through on my mother's wishes and went into accounting. This insight clarified my father's blessing and made it less ambiguous in my mind. He was telling me to go into another profession.

There you have a blessing and a curse. My father was giving me a blessing to pursue whatever profession I wanted. This was strong enough to overcome my mother's desire to see me as an accountant in his firm. I was cursed when my father told me I hate to write.

What you see here are a series of communications one can pick up that are of seminal importance to one's life. The blessing or the curse comes to have great force in an individual's life.

A blessing can work as a prophecy to be fulfilled. When you are unaware, all you can do is resign oneself to the consequences of a curse or fight a disabling, costly battle against it. You can see why I search my own existence for evidence of blessings and curses. I want to be free to choose my own life by bringing them to awareness. As you might expect, bringing the blessing and the curse to awareness made it easier for me to write and freed me to do it without physical symptoms that caused me discomfort.

Augie

PS. I will hesitate in my writing to await your comments. In the meantime—may you choose your own blessings.

Dear B. J.,

You are absolutely right. I was uptight when I wrote you
the last letters. The curse and blessing I wrote about began to
mushroom with associations and threatened to become a treatise
on my life. When we carry out a rumination this far, it becomes
a nexus and does begin to explain and give meaning to much
in life. If we see philosophy as Bergson does, crystallizing on
one idea, we may see philosophy as an extended nexus that may
begin anywhere.

I promise to lighten up this letter, and I have stifled the
Simmel-Groddeck analysis for now to return to curses. You asked
me what brought the cure and made it easier to write. I can never
be certain about the dynamics. A great weight seemed lifted when
I identified my father's curse. I understood that he probably had
forgotten his remark and did not mean it as a curse. I, the guilty
party, had picked up on his phrase because it suited my needs.
When I made further sense of his blessing and saw he was sincere
in wishing that I work in a profession other than accounting,
more pressure was released for me. I had no need to feel guilty
for leaving accounting. I felt an immediate sense of relief when
these ideas were revealed, but it took some time and constant
reminders until the shadow of the curse was lifted. Before I sat
down to write, I would remind myself of these ideas and then
proceed with my writing. Eventually I was able to forget such
reminders.

One other problem remained to be worked out, and that
was how to deal with the knowledge that it was my mother who
wanted me to go into accounting. It was quite easy to see that
in making such pronouncements she was misinterpreting my
father's desires. He did not want me to be an accountant.
Nonetheless, uneasy feelings remained with me. I thought more
about my writing habits and realized that after a certain period
of time during a writing session I would feel tired and quit, then

go home quickly to my wife. My guilt was expressed by limiting my writing sessions because they would make me seem disloyal to my wife (mother). During the summers I rarely got any professional work done because my wife was home and I felt guilty for staying away and writing. While at home, I would do household repairs alone and read all day, but I felt compelled to be there.

No, I was not confused in my writing between my wife and my mother. Only in my behavior did these transferences occur. My wife was the stand-in for my mother and a reminder that I went into the wrong profession. Overcoming this problem was far from easy. The solution took the usual form of communication. I told my wife that I felt guilty about staying away and writing. We discussed it for some time, and she said she did not mind my absence for she also is a private person and likes time to do her own reading and work. I had won release to do my work.

A key to the dynamic I describe is that my mother always protected my father by allowing nothing to interfere with his work. Anything that was illegitimate, that is, not work, she resented if my father did not spend the time with her. My writing was illegitimate (in her eyes as seen by me), and I felt guilty doing it for any extended period of time.

If I may anticipate a criticism here, you might say that my thinking is reductive, that all in this situation does not devolve from the mother. I can only report to you what I find. Your ruminations about your problems may not take you to that point. You may find no mother or father. The key is, and I made this point to you some letters back, no idiosyncrasy is without cause or association with other events in your life. The fact that I hated to write, that I would get fatigued and quit after four hours of writing, was not merely a cultural norm and natural fatigue. Nor can you take as an accident or trick of body rhythm that you can only write in the morning, at a desk, in a bright room, with a handful of sunflower seeds, at the typewriter in your study. If those are your habits and cause you no trouble, then why bother to analyze them? However, if you find yourself at a disadvantage when your office is too noisy, your sunflower seeds are missing, or your typewriter is in need of repair, then you may want to engage in it-talk.

The truly idiosyncratic we may think to analyze. As a college student I had a friend who was having difficulty with his schoolwork. He was having difficulty studying. When I pressed further, it seemed that he could only start studying on the hour or half-hour. If it was 12:01, he had to wait until 12:30 to study. What I discovered was that he found every possible diversion to keep from looking at the clock to see the hour and half-hour. Even when friends were present to "help" him, he would divert their attention until it was 12:01 or 12:31 so he had to wait another half hour. We can see something is wrong in my friend's idiosyncrasy, but in most of the Uncle-Frank habits we have, elements are equally absurd. The only difference is that my college friend could not fool others and Uncle Frank could.

I keep straying from the blessing/curse because it opens such interesting avenues of inquiry. I loved your story about your brother. He grew up with the blessing that he was a good person. Your parents constantly reminded him of this and he took this in as all important. You are correct in saying that sometimes a blessing/curse need be said only once and other times the oracle from Delphi may constantly repeat the message. What finally makes it a blessing or a curse is whether or not we accept it as such.

Your brother's case truly exemplifies where the same utterance may be taken as a blessing at times and a curse at others. When you were growing up, it kept him from getting into trouble with his friends. In your neighborhood, the likelihood was great he could have practiced a criminal career. In college, as you correctly pointed out, he worked against his image as a "good boy" by deliberately drinking too much, messing up his grades, and being arrested in numerous protest marches. Now he is back to taking the injunction as a blessing and serving as a good father and loyal employee. For him, being a "good boy" was a blessing to be lived up to and a curse to be lived down.

More generally, the blessing/curse is a *prophecy* by someone other than the recipient. We call the prophecy a blessing if it leads to consequences that the recipient views as good and a curse if it leads to consequences that the recipient rebels against and tries to live down. In my mind, both take away from freedom. I would rather understand the prophecy and free myself from its pervasive force. With this approach, there are no blessings or curses.

What interests me so much about prophecy is how it gets so quickly to central issues. My friend Groddeck or I or anyone practicing self-analysis for any length of time can begin with an itch on the face, a watch chain, or a sore knee and use it as the beginning of an association nexus to get at our lives. Even when those without training or practice are asked about prophecy, they can quickly understand it and come up with an analysis. Prophecy gives one easy access to life.

Let me give you an illustration by telling you of a brief conversation I had with a friend just yesterday. As you may gather, most of my illustrations are taken in their immediacy, for the details remain fresh to me. Many other examples could serve here. My friend, a professor at the university, and I discuss our ideas. I stopped by his house and told him I had been thinking about what I called curses. I gave him one or two examples and he began to explode with ideas. During the next hour, I scarcely uttered a sound. The word *curse* is the best entry into such discussions.

He began by telling me about an early IQ test when he was told that he had an extraordinary IQ. A few years later he was tested again and found to be average. This pattern kept repeating itself, and he became tied to these outside evaluations of his worth. This was the curse imposed upon him at an early age. As you can see, B. J., the curse often revolves about the "self worth" of the individual. The blessing/curse tells one of his or her potential or limitations. A free individual will reject these valuations of himself or herself and see that there is freedom to choose. The person blessed with great athletic ability is free only if he or she independently decides to use that gift. Such a person has character by my definition. Prophecies involve judgments of and by others, and we should stay free of these entanglements. My friend's life is tied up in these judgments. Without the objective data, the IQ tests, he is always uncertain of his own worth and the worth of others. As I have suggested in my writings, judgments about worth are inevitable yet destructive, for there are no absolute answers. There are only a multitude of standards that we can apply to ourselves.

My foregoing musings did not intrude on his thought processes. After he told me about the IQ tests that were both a blessing and a curse, he talked with me about other ideas. Finally his mind returned to the idea of curses and he said, "Now I will tell you of the curse that affected me the most." He had just returned from a high school reunion, and conversations with a former girlfriend prompted the following observations. In high school, my friend went out with this girl, whose grades were superior to his. Her home situation was not the best, and she was taken into the home of a teacher at the high school. The teacher told my friend Frank that he was NOT GOOD ENOUGH for the girl. He came from a lower class, his grades were not as good as hers, and the teacher made several similar statements to dissuade him from ever taking the girl out again. This remained a curse for him that he has been working against it all his life.

You can see the structural similarity in curses here. I mentioned to Frank that his earlier IQ curse was related to the teacher's statement. He agreed and said that the teacher's statement seemed to sum up these feelings. In other words, the curse took because he was already feeling guilty about having an average IQ. In much of our conversation that followed, he elaborated on the many influences the curse had on his life then and now.

All of this had come to full awareness at the reunion when he talked with his old girlfriend. She related that this teacher was not talented but thought of herself as elitist. She had taken over the girl's life and chased male and female from her. The teacher had memorized students' high school grades and used them as a cudgel to keep potential friends and suitors away. The girl finally rebelled and left the schoolteacher. All of this came as a great surprise and relief to my friend. He said that he felt actual physical relief when these facts were revealed. I did not pursue this, for as a friend and teacher I do not pry beyond what someone wants to give. Apparently, the relief came from knowing that this teacher was possessive, unfair, and worked the same tactics on many others. My friend acted as if a great weight had been taken off his back (often the cause of backache, though not in this case). As frequently happens, the more you explore a curse the more surprises you come up with.

I have gone on too long already, one of my foibles.

Love to your brother,

Augie

Letters to Scott

Dear Scott,

Now that you have decided to read Groddeck's *Book of the It,* I must tell you something of how to read the book. I do not mean this in a condescending way, for you have all the mental preparation necessary to read him. What is necessary is to warn you that much of what he writes can put the reader off. He is extraordinarily clever and insightful, but he is rarely read today.

Freud leads his readers gently into psychoanalysis in *Introductory Lectures.* He begins by talking of slips of the tongue and tries to understand this ubiquitous feature of social life. Only later, after he has the reader hooked, does he introduce his more radical ideas. By then, Freud's argument has become compelling for the reader.

Contrast Freud's approach with Groddeck's. In the first letter in his *Book of the It,* Groddeck tells the reader that he hates science. In the next few letters, he informs the reader that there are male pregnancies and mother hate. Later on in the book, before a particularly important argument, he discusses anal intercourse. No wonder Groddeck is not read! Before the reader has developed any sympathy with him, he is offending his or her sensibilities and overturning cherished beliefs. All of this takes place without adequate preparation for the reader. It is an abrupt intimacy to read his book, almost a breach of etiquette. As you know, such obstacles never bother me, so I quickly plunged on. I hope you do the same.

I mentioned to you before that Groddeck knew himself well, so you might justifiably ask what he was doing by turning his readers off. The activity of subverting one's own efforts I have come to describe as "shooting oneself in the foot." In letter twenty-eight, near the end of his book, Groddeck indicates that he is aware of this propensity in himself. He describes the phenomenon of one's it giving off negative impressions to another whose attentions one would like to capture. Before a big date, boys and girls often break out in zits, spots, pimples, blemishes, whiteheads, etc. Their hands may sweat. Their breath may be bad or their underarms wet. Groddeck feels that if we are not sure whether our affection is to be returned by the other person, in order to find out, we create a condition that is likely to put that person off. What we have here for Groddeck is a test of affection. We know that the person really likes us if he or she can put up with the spots, bad breath, sweaty palms, or running nose. Groddeck says little more about what I call shooting oneself in the foot, but he hints that this occurs in his writing. He is worried about "oppressive angels" who will read his text looking for errors.

Let me complete his analysis and give some examples of my own, then this matter of Groddeck's propensity to discourage the reader might be clear. Groddeck, throughout his writings, speaks of his indifference towards writing and caring whether he is ever read. He proclaims that he does not want disciples, that practice is his first priority, and that one can always read the master, Freud. Groddeck, in his own terms, protests too much.

There is much evidence to show that Groddeck wanted his materials published and that he craved recognition from Freud and others. His letters to Freud are replete with these anxieties. He was unsure of the sympathies of his audience. Would they like his works or not? When we are not sure of people's affections, we provide them with the ammunition to dislike us. Groddeck decided to publish his letters without correction, without toning down the language or sexual references. Since the oppressive angels were going to scrutinize him closely, he was going to show them the flaws straight out. I believe that shooting himself in the foot in this way curtailed his readership greatly. Freud sensed this tendency and chided Groddeck for pressing his antiscientific public stance. Freud suggested to Groddeck that his views of science were not as radical as his public stance. Although Groddeck partially understood why he was sabotaging his own work, he nevertheless proceeded to do so. We will never know whether he was fully aware of the extent to which he sabotaged his own work; whether he knew it but could not overcome the tendency; or whether he felt it was not worth the effort to please his audience. But whatever his proclivities, Groddeck is well worth reading.

I want to speak a little more about the idea of shooting yourself in the foot, for it is a common tendency. The it is setting up a test to see if others really are in sympathy with you. When I was first going out with your mother, I remember feeling quite ill at ease at her house. I was not the polite, perfect person her family was seeing. They seemed (this is a key word) to like me, and I remember walking very carefully around their house, afraid to damage or bump into anything. One day I picked up a large flat decorative plate that was a favorite of your grandmother's. I broke it into thousands of tiny pieces. I use language advisedly here. The plate did not slip. Someone did not distract me. I smashed the plate. I cannot recall exactly how it happened, but I get visual images of holding the plate up and releasing it to smash on the concrete. I know my it did it deliberately. Most vivid at the time were my feelings. I felt this enormous sense of relief, and an irrepressible smile appeared on my face that I tried to turn to an embarrassed smile—but it was one of pure pleasure. Take me or leave me now. I smash plates and do all sorts of negative things. Do you still like me?

I could describe a million ways I shoot myself in the foot. For example, I never give a maximum effort to anything. I hold something in reserve. Although this looks like a different attitude altogether, it is a variant of the same principle. Holding back is an excuse, an answer to those who find me wanting. I can always say, "If they don't like this, I am able to do better." What I have built in here is a double protection. If you see my faults and still have sympathies with me, you have passed the test. If my faults put you off, then your judgment may not ultimately be correct because I can do better.

Other people have provided me with numerous examples of built-in protection. One friend of mine writes in an obscure style, another pads his writing with unnecessary detail. Many people "play hurt"—they announce that they performed despite a bad ankle, wrote while suffering with a headache, achieved under poor working conditions. Bringing these ideas to light gives me a choice. When I ask colleagues to critique my work now, I ask them how I am shooting myself in the foot. Then

I can choose to follow their instructions and excise or add certain items. Believe me, we all strain to do our "best."

O.K. I will get around to it. What is a letter from one's father but an object lesson? We have discussed these matters before, and I feel you shoot yourself in the foot. You will not show your work to others until it is "perfect." Of course this makes working difficult, and now you can see why. You are trying to do your "best," but the risks are very great. There is little recourse when someone critiques your work. The critic can sense defensiveness in your work, the building in of invulnerability. In the role of critic, one is *supposed* to find mistakes. Whether mistakes are there or not, the critic is obliged to find some, and your defenses are shattered.

I had a student once who began to get all As in college and he developed fears. He was on the verge of dropping out of school, paranoid about instructors who could sabotage his grades. I told him to make it his business to get a B, because trying to build invulnerability was costing him his equilibrium. He was about to retire from college because of difficulties in dealing with others. He would return to the admiration and sympathy of his parents. I did not see it all that clearly then, but the advice I gave was correct. He got his B and successfully completed his undergraduate degree.

Now I can tell you one of the ways I most often shoot myself in the foot. When I teach, I always have the tendency to keep the class past the end of the period. I keep saying, "One more minute," which gets the students mentally prepared to leave, and then I keep them on. I thought that this warning let them know I was not prepared to keep them in class forever. When I began thinking about what I was doing, I realized I was testing their patience. They stay a minute, and then I tack on another minute. The same is true of my conversations with people. I can clearly read cues as to when people want to take leave, and then I engage them in one more bit of dialogue. The same is true of my writing; I try people's patience.

What I am doing is testing their sympathies. In one of the first classes I taught, I remember my let-down feeling when the students slapped their books together and took their bored-neutral faces to the next class. Even though I had been a student most of my life, it seemed appropriate that my students applaud. In other words, whether I am in conversation or in front of a class, I am unsure of the sympathies of my audience. My encores allow me to see if they like me enough to stay, even though I have violated their freedom to leave the room.

It is no coincidence that I remember a book by Francis Wellman, a turn-of-the-century lawyer, who wrote *The Art of Cross-Examination.* His favorite principle was to allow the audience, in this case the jury, to discover things for themselves. If they think they have made the discovery, they will be more inclined to your side. Do not overkill the obvious. Similarly, my graduate school advisor spoke of not fulfilling every idea the student wants to hear. Leave them hungry. No wonder I remember these maxims. They appeal to my I. Yet my it fights against these ideas. "If I overkill with information, do you still love me?"

So we have my letter as demonstrating the same principle. You are quick and capable, and all I had to do was tell you about the shooting of oneself in the foot as it relates to Groddeck. You could then choose or not to analyze yourself. I went for overkill and so I violated another principle: making an analysis for another person. Knowing all this, I let the letter stand. With a son, overkill or underkill, fathers are rarely heeded—and vice versa. This is a good enough rationalization for me to let this letter remain as it is. My propensity is to overkill.

Love,

Dad

PS. Going to the doctor to have a bullet removed from my foot.

Dear Scott,

I was interested to hear that you decided to read Groddeck and continued to read on despite some important objections. As you know, I have thought a great deal about his writings. What I will try to do is to meet your objections and suggest how I have tried to handle them. You raise too many of them, many novel ones that I have not thought about. My answers will come in due course. Given your inquiring mind, I am sure that neither Groddeck nor I will satisfy you. All I hope is that you may view us with enough sympathy that some fraction of his or my views may be of some use to you. More likely, you and I will merely shape up our separate views. Either way, the dialogue will be useful to me and I hope to you.

You object to the way in which he uses symbols, so here is as good a place as any to start. Before I answer your criticisms, let me give you a description of his views, many of which are taken from his essay "The Compulsion to Use Symbols." Groddeck believes we think always in symbols on the unconscious level (in this essay he uses Freud's not his own terminology). As an example, he says that when we move about the house we meet symbols at every step and each one suggests another. Groddeck borrowed the idea of the symbol from Goethe's writings. Emerson saw the symbol in every manifestation of "nature," and Groddeck broadens Emerson's idea of nature to all the objects we confront in life. The symbol for Groddeck is an object that stands for another.

Not only do we interpret stimuli through symbols, but we express ourselves the same way. Groddeck (again using Freud's language—this time making the distinction between mind and body) says that neurosis as well as the organic symptom is a symbolic stirring of the unconscious. In all of our overt gestures, including language, our behavior is symbolic. The task remains for us to understand this language, whether it be verbal or nonverbal.

136

Groddeck uses the concepts of the unconscious and repression to describe why this language is better understood by the child. Adults repress much that is in the unconscious, but children, who are freer of repression, have more access to this material. Groddeck sees that common sense, which for him is stupidity brought on by repression, replaces the earlier intuition of the child. The adult has to discipline himself or herself to understand this hidden language.

In an earlier article in *Imago,* Groddeck put forth the idea that human languages had their inception in the erotic drives of the unconscious. The very sounds of languages express erotic feelings. Moreover, in most of his analyses, symbols have erotic connotations. Much like Freud, Groddeck believed in the universality of some symbols. Often he makes no differentiation between those symbolic associations that he has made and those which he shares with other people. No doubt, some associations we all share. This is obvious to him in his analysis of literature— Goethe, Peer Gynt, the Ring Cycle, fables, nursery rhymes, and other tales.

Now I believe I am ready to deal with your objections. You do not think that we always express ourselves through the symbol. A full reading of *The Book of the It* may break through this objection as you let go and begin to allow yourself to relax and free associate. Groddeck's it-talk will begin to force you to think in these modes and bring you to awareness of how these processes work.

I have begged the question, sending you back to Groddeck. I must try, however difficult, to directly address your question. Perhaps I can do it best by showing how I first took a public stand on the issue of the symbol, a stand not unlike your own. In high school, I began to disavow anything but a literal interpretation of art, poetry, or story. All of this came to a climax when my class went to a museum of art in New York City. Upon our arrival, the teacher drew us around her in front of a picture, one that presumably struck her fancy, and asked the class, "What do you see?" Her breast swelled with what seemed to me was a false sensibility as she asked the question with Olympian superiority. Not normally the wise guy or class clown, I chose to answer her. With finality and conviction in my voice, I said,

"I see a horse." Taken aback, she asked, hoping I suppose that someone else would answer, "And what else do you see?" Quickly I answered, more definitely and loudly, "A horse, nothin' else." With a few more parries, she was crushed; the class was won to my position; and the teacher's trip was ruined. The museum was, at the time, the one place where a teenager had access to the female anatomy. So, for me the trip was a triumph and a joy.

I tell you this story because it lays out the positivism that I formally accepted as a graduate student and that allowed me to close off from awareness thoughts of symbol, metaphor, and association. Also, I can try to reconstruct for you why I accepted positivism. For me, and possibly some of my classmates, the acceptance of poetry, art, and opera was tantamount to an admission you were gay. I shut the door that day to any ideas that I might have such ambivalent feelings about myself, an ambivalence, as Groddeck suggests, we all share. A horse is a horse. Also there is an acceptance of the purposive literal world of the adult who has no time for dreaming, fantasy, or any other childhood activity. What I saw was a horse. You could look at it stand in place, ride it if you lived out West, or eat it if you lived in France. The picture I saw was a horse standing, no more no less.

Why did I choose to take my stand on the picture of a horse? Was it because it was the first picture we came upon and I was already geared for my comment, no matter the object? I do not think so! Why then on this trip and not at the opera or while reading Shakespeare's *Macbeth* in class? I believe it was because of the horse. I felt great ambivalence towards horses. At summer camp, my parents paid an extra fifty dollars so that I could ride horses, and I remember my fears. Horror stories abounded. Riding a horse, drowning in the lake, or contracting polio were the three ways we could lose our lives at camp. The latter two I could do little about, other than hugging the shore while swimming. Riding the horse was optional, but my parents would have wasted the money if I had not ridden. I survived the summer but came away with ambivalent feelings towards horses. Horses were devils. They were stupid and disobedient. They were devilish and clever (just look in their eyes). They were graceful and clumsy, had a distinct smell, were receptacles for flies, had the biggest penises I had seen on a living thing, and seemed to be in pain with bits in their mouths. I could go on and on, but will stop for the sake of brevity.

Why did I ride in the first place? As children we played cowboys and Indians, and each of us kept a favorite horse. My favorite was Silver. Palominos were far less masculine. My friends could ride Roy Roger's Trigger, but I would ride the Lone Ranger's masculine stud. We were the horses' masters. We could run away, charge others, and fight; the horse would only accelerate our speed and impact. The horse was our friend and companion. Horses in the stories I read were wild and free. Tamed they were servants of man's freedom. No wonder I attempted to ride at camp and convinced my parents to pay the fifty dollars. What do I remember about the rides? Never walk behind the horse; always mount from the left side, the Western saddle at least had the pedicle to hang onto; and get the oldest horse to ride.

A long story and set of associations, I know. But now you understand why I gave my literal answer to the picture. I protested too much. Not only did I have a thousand associations with horses, as we do with everything else, but these associations were fresh, vivid, and tinged with strong feelings of freedom, death, and unreason. Although I see much in a horse, on that day I chose to say little.

That day fixed me for quite a time as a positivist. I was comfortable in an adult mode, denied all sorts of problematic associations, and could reach consensual agreement with many in our culture. But you can see that now I agree with Groddeck that we think in terms of symbols. Perhaps if you try such a mental exercise—take a thought in which you feel the symbol plays no part and analyze it—you will change your mind.

Although you are not a positivist, I think you will find interesting how positivism is, in Groddeck's terms, a systematic repression. Gustav Bergmann suggests a correspondence between reality and the concept. We may define a horse as a four-legged creature that eats hay and neighs. This horse we may observe running, jumping, kicking, eating oats, drinking water, and having intercourse. Or we might define a horse as an animal that is fifteen hands high; has pointed ears, a mane, and four legs; and runs faster than a sheep. Then we may see what other activities are related to a horse. What are we doing here? Publicly, we are deciding how to agree on what a horse is by using associations that do not evoke strong associations. A horse is not an animal with a much bigger penis than a man's or a menace to children under foot. After we have defined a horse, then we identify definite patterns in a horse, ones everyone can observe.

What a way to tame and (excuse the pun) bridle one's symbolic associations. How much better to tame associations of their emotive content and bring them into agreement with the complacent definition of the concept. The adult world is not one of dreams and symbols, but one of agreement. Yes, for the positivist there are symbols and associations, but they are shared with others and controlled through conscious thoughts. The child in us is relegated to creativity—to make a wild association, to suggest a new avenue of inquiry. Creativity for the positivist is not a process that is going on all the time below awareness but a gift, a muse that (once in a while) can contribute. The positivist expends most of his or her efforts making ties between agreed upon symbols that have been drained of emotive contents.

I know that you are not a positivist, but the implications of holding to the idea that we are not primarily symbolizing animals tends to imply that position. For now, I, the father, am the child and you, the son, are the adult.

Next letter I will conclude my comments on the symbol and your objections.

Love,

Dad Bad Glad Sad

Dear Scott,

This letter should be easier to write because I am in basic
agreement with you on your criticism of Groddeck. You are not
so certain of the importance of childhood sexuality even though
you understand that Freud and Groddeck meant by sex more
than the sex act. Groddeck, in his analysis, finds Oedipus, the
castration complex, voluptuousness and sexuality in women giving birth, as well as many other manifestations of childhood sexuality. Groddeck speaks of how masturbation is prior to intercourse and continues into old age. If we do not believe him on
these ideas, we are asked to go to a zoo and watch children
watching the monkeys. Then we will be convinced about the
importance of sexuality.

Groddeck was much influenced by Freud in these matters,
and both men fought against strict sexual taboos which no longer
shock. Your generation, most of all, seems to have fewer inhibi-
tions about sex. What do we do then with Groddeck's views?
We may now look dispassionately at the issue and decide. We
could take the easy way out and say that the Victorian's neuroses
were more tied up than ours with sexuality because this was the
forbidden yet desirable drive of the age. Therefore, what
Groddeck found is not what I would find, but both of us are
right in our respective time frame.

Groddeck is inconsistent on this issue as on other issues
where he assumes Freud's views. At times, he speaks of the
universality of sexuality, as when he speaks of the origins of symbols. He is eager in his writings to agree with Freud, and this
is one area where Freud broke with many of his colleagues. Much
of Groddeck's writing was undoubtedly meant to please Freud,
and the idea of the universality of sexuality would undoubtedly
please him. Groddeck did not distort his data and found that
sexuality was overwhelmingly important. Nonetheless, there are
many times when Groddeck does not speak of sexuality or link

141

it to selfishness, power, fears, or many other phenomena. He never posits for the it an eros, pleasure principle, or any singular motive or instinct. The it is life and multifarious. Groddeck's idea of the it and organic illness do not stand or fall on the importance of sexuality.

As we find many times in Groddeck, he borrows ideas from Freud and does not fully integrate them into his own theory. Freud's ideas expanded Groddeck's thought and led Groddeck to help many patients. For Groddeck, the question of the universality of sex was an empirical one and not a logical correlate of his theory. He found sexuality very widespread, but if he did not find it, nothing would happen to his theory.

Your objection was that in expanding your own awareness, sexuality was not ubiquitous. In my own analyses, I tend to find it more often. I find old Oedipus, as well as confirming some other structures Groddeck and Freud found. What we are speaking of here is an empirical investigation, and it is best to enter into it without preconceived notions. We may find Oedipus because we are looking for him; or we may find organ inferiority, or archetypes, or other structures for the same reason. I know that this is what the "classical" psychoanalysts fought so bitterly about. Your objections to what Groddeck has found are well taken. You may find something very different. Groddeck may find different results empirically than you do, but you can accommodate yourself comfortably to his framework. As for me, I tend to find in myself and others much of what Groddeck finds. This is not because it is necessary to the theory. Perhaps I want to please the master; or more likely, his examples interfere with my own associations and lead me to certain conclusions. I hope I have developed checks against this tendency but perhaps not. Do your analysis and tell me what you find. Please remember that I sympathize with Groddeck and do much to construct him favorably. Read and interpret him for yourself without my mediation.

Your final objection to the symbol is right on the mark. Groddeck tends to find a symbol and assume the meaning would be the same for another person. This is a flaw found in the thinking of most psychoanalysts of Groddeck's time. We are all too familiar with the tall building, the lake, the train going through the tunnel, the sensation of flying, and other symbols that find their way even into mass entertainment. These symbols are used as guideposts in analysis, shortcuts to understanding.

There is danger in interpretation if we assume the universality of symbols. This danger is when the friend, therapist, or critic links the meaning of a term you use with a "universal" symbol. In other words, free associating, for them, becomes the search for universal symbols.

Perhaps I can show you the absurd lengths this can go to in literary criticism. The critic is often guessing at the associations that the author is making. The critic assumes that if he makes the connection the author must have made it as well. Robert Penn Warren gave an example of this when he commented on a scholarly article written about one of his stories. The critic pointed out that the street sign that Warren refers to in the story bears a girl's first name and the sign for the intersecting street carries a last name. Together, the signs make up the name of a minor character in *Tess of the D'Urbervilles.* From this linkage, the critic concludes Warren's story is allegorically linked to Hardy's novel, and he discusses this theme at length in his article. Because the street signs stand for the name of a minor character in *Tess,* Warren wrote an allegory about *Tess.* Warren said he did read *Tess* when he was young, but there were no ties to *Tess* in his story. Warren took the names of the streets from signs on the corner of the block on which he lived.

We cannot presume the universality of symbols. Let us see the degree to which Groddeck does this, and whether there is any basis for it. In his writings, Groddeck rarely says whether the imagery is universal or idiosyncratic. Sometimes he may say that the rat resembles the sausage and that the seeds, like sperm, break out of the cucumber. He appears to be trying to convince the reader of the generalizability of the symbol. No doubt he is appealing to the reader for the universality of the symbol. When he is careful, however, he speaks of the it as truth; truth being the way the it, without guile, associates one idea with the other. We can take Groddeck's approach two ways: he pushes the universality of a symbol or tries to show us how the individual is a creative symbolizing person. I treat Groddeck in the latter fashion and feel that only the student, patient, or author can ultimately tell what the connection is between one object and another.

I feel that Groddeck was pushing both purposes, not carefully differentiating between them. There are some merits to speaking of universal or near universal symbols. When you are with some friends, look at the clouds passing overhead. Often you and they will agree on configurations when there are strong resemblances to another object. I see a clown or a fish or the face of a woman framed by hair. As we know from the drawing of two women as seen from different perspectives, we make the associations, and even perfect isomorphism will not necessarily bring the same association. When Groddeck speaks of a patient who remembers falling and breaking her arm, he asks her what she saw at the time. She answers, "Asparagus in the window." We go, aha! The sight of a penis makes her have a moral fall and she breaks her arm. In fact, this is what did happen to her. We tend to generalize when we see such obvious isomorphism. Groddeck is not beyond that temptation. Many times we can guess right. Many times we may be wrong.

What also helps to make for the possibility of universals are culturally agreed upon symbols. A culture assigns to words meanings that we can agree on, and we agree that certain symbols stand for other symbols. In our vocabulary we have many words for physical objects that have become associated with parts of the anatomy. We all laugh as we think of nuts, balls, and chops. General use in the culture of the public symbol gives us consciously thought of associations. Whether truly general to the it or not, when a director or novelist uses certain "symbols," we all go, aha! We know what he or she is referring to—the "Freudian symbol." Hence, knowledge of psychoanalysis gives us common associations we can identify in the literature and the mass media.

There is much temptation to generalize because of isomorphism, culturally acknowledged symbols, and popular knowledge of psychoanalysis. We feel we can understand for someone else. Groddeck does this as much as you or I. In my own work, I try to keep free of generalizations about the importance of sexuality and the contents of the it, but like Groddeck I am prey to such a weakness. I see sympathy as important as well as the idea of the curse, rumination, and the nexus. All of these should be taken as methodological suggestions; do not see them if they are not there. There is a tenuous line between telling people what they might expect to find and convincing them that they see it. As a philosopher, I say expand awareness and look at symbols anew, but I am not above giving people a peek at generalized contents.

Again, Groddeck's philosophy is not predicated on finding generalized symbols. On the contrary, he suggests the it is rich and clever in its associations. At one point, he says that all symbols can be male and female. For instance, a cucumber can be the penis with sperm or the uterus with eggs. This remark alone suggests that universality in symbols is not possible. Even if we culturally define words and relate one object to another, the it may have other ideas. My I suggested there is universal agreement as to what a horse is. Yet, my it, to use Groddeck's term, was far from agreement. The it is far too clever to be bound by cultural agreement. To me a horse is a devil, freedom, death, and many other associations.

Let me give you an example about how clever we are as symbolizing animals. I will give you a nursery rhyme and you see what your associations are. This is how I remember it.

> Four and twenty blackbirds
> Baked in a pie;
> When the pie was opened,
> the birds began to sing.
> Isn't this a dainty dish
> to bring before the king?

If you have made your associations, here are mine. This was a significant rhyme for me. The king is the father and the pie is the chest-stomach area. When the pie was opened, it was rotten, and the birds were evidence of the rot. As the pie, I felt ashamed at being exposed as rotten before the king (my father). No matter if you have the same interpretation. I told this story to a friend and she said that the birds singing meant liberation to her. So you see, we can have multiple interpretations strongly felt. My temptation here would be to guess how you reacted, for there is always great temptation to generalize. My disposition is to resist, but I cannot always. So it is with such matters.

Those are my views on the symbol and I await your comments.

Love,

Dad

Dear Scott,

I can appreciate that you want some more time to think about symbols before you answer my letters. Yes, I agree that Groddeck never fully answered questions about epidemics and the inevitability of disease. Durrell is correct on this point. In a speech to the Spring Valley Medical School, which I enclose, I speak of the rationale of using cause interna as a working hypothesis. This will help you some in understanding my position, but I should elaborate in this letter about the epidemic.

In my first year of college, the "Asian flu" began to affect the student body. Large numbers of students were hospitalized, and the dorms were turned into hospital wards. This was the first year that anyone of my generation could remember flu hitting so many people with such magnitude and seriousness. Nobody seemed to be exempt. I remember watching other people catch the flu and thinking, I am next. One day I came home from basketball practice and told my roommate that I thought I was coming down with it. We all talked about the flu constantly, searched incessantly for symptoms, and assiduously tried to avoid those who manifested symptoms. Hank, my roommate and boyhood friend, looked at me during one such conversation, and I remember that I had expected sympathy from him and an acknowledgment that he and I would come down with the flu next. Instead he abruptly said, "I will not get it." That was the end of the conversation. Of course, I came down with the flu the next day; and although everyone else I knew caught it, Hank never did.

This encounter was often on my mind in years to come. Hank denied he would get the flu with such confidence and finality that I could not forget it. We had no vaccines then, and he had no ideas of immunity or prior record of having the flu. When I opened the Groddeck book, this was one of the first episodes I remembered. Interpretations would be that he was immune,

147

he was never exposed, or he was just plain lucky. If I may try my hand at another interpretation, he manifested no reason for getting it, no fear of the disease as well. The virus was around, but he was not going to catch it. My other friends and I went out and caught it, perhaps for different reasons. The fear of catching the flu and the suspense were almost too much. I remember feeling relief when I finally came down with it. The suspense was over; and just as important, if I caught it earlier rather than later, I could have the Thanksgiving vacation to rest up. The season was rainy, and we were "chilled" coming home from basketball practice everyday with wet heads exposed to cold. That is why, in our minds, we caught it.

While I look for cause interna, most people search for the cause externa. The weather, pollen, change in temperature, foods, too few vitamins, even phases of the moon cause our ailments. We explain our illnesses all the time in an ex-post facto way. Other times, when we expect to fall victim to an epidemic, we look for the "evil signs" that predict our own illness. As well, we see all those about us getting sympathy from others: relatives are being summoned, strangers are solicitous. The pressures of being a first-year student are great and disease immobilizes us, so that for the first time since entering college we have no responsibility for grades. (We know that we might have to work doubly hard to catch up in schoolwork; that, however, is not the it but the I, or awareness, speaking.) There was a flu virus, and for me (but not for my roommate), there were plenty of reasons to go out and catch the flu. I know that almost everyone would consciously deny wanting to catch the flu. We had high fevers, were immobilized, and felt terrible; and symptoms could last for a week or more. The it makes the association between illness and sympathy, illness and rest, illness and perhaps guilt at remaining well. The it does not weigh all the factors and then make a reasoned choice to stay well. This is a key idea to bear in mind. Our awareness rarely ever demands to be sick. Here rests the resistance of others to Groddeck's ideas.

My example took place long ago, and I cannot be certain of exactly what happened. All I can do is show you a plausible explanation as to why we can have epidemics, and yet the diseases are not inevitable for us as individuals. None of my concerns and perceptions seemed to affect my roommate. He was confident and determined that he would not get sick. Perhaps he stopped illness on the level of will; his awareness so harnessed his life that illness was not entertained. In a similar situation, I asked a friend of mine whether he ever made himself ill. He has traveled to Tanzania, Somalia, and European countries extensively. He said, "No, I don't make myself ill, but I am darn well sure that I won't get sick when I travel to foreign countries." When he returns, however, he inevitably comes down with exotic diseases.

Before we settle on will as an explanation, we must be somewhat careful. Most people profess a determination not to get sick. In my examples of Hank and the flu as well as of my world-traveler friend, perhaps they could find no reason to be ill. My world-traveler friend admitted that when he returns home ill there is comfort for all the hardship and work while abroad. So, I am not sure whether will (that is, the ascension of awareness over the it) prevents illness.

Perhaps you find me too tentative here, but I do not want to go further than existing evidence. All I am trying to do is point out the plausibility of avoiding the epidemic. Before I close my case, look at some of the studies in collective behavior. Here you will find documented cases of physical symptoms shown simultaneously by many people, including skin eruptions, fever, chills, vomiting, and so forth, with no "physical cause."

As for my own participation in the epidemic, I gave you many reasons why I may have chosen to come down with the flu. I am not positive which was the necessary or sufficient reason; I recall all of them as concerns. Everything was there from the need for social conformity to an excuse for seeing my girlfriend (your mom). I can guess that the most important reason was catching the flu early so I had the vacation to recover.

What the epidemic illustrates is that the reasons for catching a disease are individual. One person may have been told that he has a low immunity response and is susceptible to anything; another may get ill anytime a sibling gets ill because she feels guilty about being well; another may be looking for a convenient illness and contagion suggests one; or yet another may want to get the inevitable over with. I have found all of these possibilities in people.

Let me give you a few examples of susceptibility. When I went to Florida with your sister to visit the grandparents, she came back with strep throat. My throat began to hurt and I tried to analyze why. All of the reasons I just mentioned came to mind, but they were forced, not my reasons at the time. Finally I asked myself what the consequence would be of getting a sore throat. I had asked the question earlier, but to no avail. This time the thought that occurred to me was that I would have to go to the doctor for a throat culture. Quickly I saw that I felt guilty for not having made an appointment to see my physician for my periodic checkup. He would be angry with me. Of course, I could avoid his seeing me when I went in for a throat culture, then once in the office complex, I would make an appointment to see him. When I realized the dynamics, I immediately called the doctor to make an appointment for my periodic checkup. The relief I felt was enormous; the next day my sore throat was gone. As a sidelight, I realized that when we worry about a sore throat, we self-consciously swallow, rub our tongue on the back of our throat, cough, and generally irritate our throat. The "bug" may be there; we rub it in.

So you see, the reason why one "catches" a disease from another is not the same for one person as another, nor necessarily the same reason for a person in two separate illnesses. If you think about such matters, you need not think about epidemics, but merely catching a disease or an injury from another. The first question I ask myself if I manifest any symptom is whether or not I have read or heard about a similar symptom. I have picked up symptoms of a terminally ill patient from a movie; a sore knee, tight calf muscle, and a sore back from reading about the Denver Broncos; and a stuffed nose from speaking to someone with one. Most of the time such recognition releases me from the symptom. At other times, as in the case of the sore throat, it is more complicated. Many times the reason for me is the same, but I will not tell you here. It would probably not be your reason and might confuse my main point; we are clever and individual in our illnesses.

I wish that I could give you one reason why we "catch" illness and injury from others. The best I can do is to say that the illness of another gives the it a possibility. What a great idea! What a plausible opportunity! I am tempted to say that we feel sorry for the other person who is ill and empathize with him, or resent or desire the sympathy she is getting. We have feelings about that person and the disease. The it may use both pieces of information, or as in the case of my sore throat, only the illness was important, not who had it or how I felt about her.

Let me finish with the story of a friend who just popped in to visit. He went to a doctor for an infected toe and the nurse said to him, "You're lucky you don't have the virus going around." The next day he caught it.

If you feel ill after reading this letter, or anytime in the future, ask yourself where you caught it.

Love,

Dad

Dear Scott,

Let us see if I can deal with some of the objections you raised in your letter. Why would we prefer to catch a debilitating flu when the consequences of not catching it are less severe? You are raising an interesting question, one which puzzles many people. Why not go to a party rather than endure stomach cramps? Why break a leg if you do not want to participate in sports? Why get a sore throat just so you can make a doctor's appointment? Awareness is not at issue here, Scott, but rather thoughts below the level of awareness. All of our illnesses or injuries are solutions to what is bothering us, but what you object to is that they seem so extreme, indirect, and absurd at times. Once we understand that to our awareness these solutions seem ridiculous, and we accept this fact, then we can help ourselves.

The illnesses or injuries are often extreme. They might even be life threatening if the ultimate response could be measured. Let me give you an example of a solution and see if I can speculate as to its magnitude. I was running the other day with a friend, and he asked me about the plans of a mutual friend. Just as I told him some information I probably should not have divulged, my foot found a rock and I almost went sprawling. Since we were on a rocky mountain path, I could have been pretty badly scraped up. First, in this example, came the violation of a trust. Next, if I had been fully aware of the situation, I might have realized that this was a minor confidence and that my running partner would never give it away. And if he did, there would be no consequences of note. My it's solution was extreme, even the inconvenience of just tripping for the crime. If I had fallen, the consequences could have been even greater.

The it has a different sense of importance than awareness has. To me, this transgression was serious; violations of confidence have always been a fear of mine. The possibility of having to face the one who entrusted me with his plans would be difficult. If I faced him with an injury, he would feel sympathy, not outrage. To the it, almost anything would seem better than to face the potential embarrassment of the situation. Direct communication with another is a most difficult situation to face. So you can see that to the it a scraped knee, even a badly twisted ankle, is preferable to facing the friend whose confidence you violated.

Can we say that the solution is extreme? Awareness that we bring to the problem may be mere deception. We may say that nothing would come of a confrontation with a friend, yet relationships are fragile. We may ruminate the whole day on how our betrayal might reach the ears of our friend. What may be in question here is whether physical pain from a scrape or bruise may be worse than enduring an interpersonal conflict. A severely bruised ankle might heal quicker than a friendship. A stomachache may be preferable to bad company. When I began my answer to you, I thought I would merely rely on the idea that our it is working without all the information, and hence I fell into the rational-awareness/irrational-it perspective. When I looked carefully, the it may be correct and awareness working on deception. As I now look at the examples, we do not have an easy answer. Physical pain may be easier to endure than that which comes from damaged relationships.

Before I close this part of the discussion, let me offer a few more considerations. Can the it measure the magnitude of responses? Did I only trip and not fall because this transgression was not great? I remember struggling mightily not to fall as I was going down. At some other time I might have given in to falling more easily. For the most part, there appears to be some symmetry. If my transgression was terrible, perhaps I would have broken my leg.

Duration of an illness or injury is often keyed to the solution of problems. One's stomach usually recovers quickly after the decision not to attend or to leave a party is irrevocably made. If I get a headache watching a game on TV, it disappears quickly when I see that your mom is no longer angry at me for watching. A sprained ankle may keep you from going on a camping trip and mend easily once you decide not to go. Often the same illness occurs when one is faced with recurrent problems.

Symptoms appear and disappear like clockwork. The predict-ability of deviation is more evidence that our illness is somewhat measured and calculated.

What is also bothersome about the physical injury or illness is how indirect a communication it is. Why not simply prepare to tell my friend that I gave away a confidence and I am sorry? Or ignore people at a party whom I do not want to talk to? We learn indirect responses at an early age. I believe some people more than others use physical illness to get their way in the world. As I explained once in an article, some may use violence, while others may devise strategies we have not even discussed. All this is understandable when we think of the child's predica-ment before he or she has adequate language skills. The infant cries and is picked up. This is similar to the infant saying, "You denied me food and I am no longer sure of your love. Before you leave me alone in the crib, tell me you love me." Even when language skills are adequate, the illness may be more effective. Can a six-year-old convince a parent that he or she does not want to go to school for any one of a number of reasons? A stomach-ache or sore throat is far more effective.

We may learn this indirect way of communicating when we lack verbal skills. More importantly, however, although an ill-ness may not be a manifestation of candor with another person, it may be far more effective in achieving the desired result. The child with the stomachache will be allowed to stay home from school; the person with the sore knee will elicit sympathy from his friend.

What I am suggesting is that what initially looks so extreme, indirect, and absurd, upon a closer look seems like an intelligent choice by the it. What makes it seem so absurd in the first place is incurring a painful injury or illness to circumvent what seems to another—or even to yourself—a minor slight, jealousy, or dif-ference of opinion. You should beware of your intense feeling that you have not brought fully to awareness. Perhaps you would rather break a leg than to go to your cousin's birthday party, get a sore throat than talk to your mother about grades, or have a sneezing attack than tell the waitress the service was bad. In conversations, you will often hear such statements said in jest.

Look at the consequences of an illness, then you will see that there is always a purpose. An actor may lose a leg to avoid failure on the stage, the artist may go blind to keep her in her studio, the writer may fall mortally ill to be appreciated for his life and work. You might not go to such extremes, but for those individuals, the solutions are of appropriate magnitude to bring the desired results and are not absurd. The difference lies in making such admissions to yourself.

Implicit in your comments about the strangeness of our bringing on our own illnesses is the plausibility of other explanations, the cause externa. Remember, I do not deny that we use external causes to our own advantage—catching colds and tripping on rocks—but these are not causes; they are handmaidens to our actions.

Listen sometime to friends explaining their illnesses. They now begin to sound absurd to me. John Vincent wakes up in the morning and is careful not to stretch too quickly for fear of pulling a muscle. He gets up and takes extra vitamin C for he fears a sore throat coming on. He curses the fact that he spent time with his friend yesterday who had a sore throat. John takes an extra glass of milk because a lot has been said on the news about bone deterioration in old age. The weather has changed today and that always seems to make his postnasal drip worse. The glare of the sun bothers him too; perhaps he should get sunglasses with UV screen. No onions on the hamburger at lunch because he has to attend a meeting and he does not want to be gassy. Perhaps that new cologne is causing a rash on his face; maybe he should try another kind. Now it is time to go out and run. He walks up the first hill for if he tries to run up it, his calf will tighten up. When his knees are warm, they will stop hurting. John remembers as a child his knees hurting at a time when he grew quickly. On a tractor as a kid, he would have to stop and stand up because of these sore knees. His father could not say much, for his arthritis made him pause often from his farm work. Dinnertime and he does not want to eat too much because it will make him sleepy. Definitely no sweets before bed or he will not go to sleep easily. He eats carbohydrates for dinner because he is running tomorrow. Before bed he puts on "MASH" because if he does not watch it or stays up later, he cannot fall asleep. He turns over on his side so he will not awaken with a stiff back in the morning.

I am sure you have heard or experienced all of these responses to external stimuli. In fact, most people, if you filter out other messages they are giving and receiving, have far more of these thoughts in their day. Does this sound any less absurd than my recourse to cause interna? Tomorrow I will write and tell you how I respond to such musings. I must sign off now because the light is dim, my stomach is growling with hunger, my arm is tired, and my foot fell asleep.

Love,

Dad

Dear Scott,

Now that you have thought about John Vincent and his troubles, I can give you my reaction to him. He is a fictional person; a composite of complaints I have heard from others in the past two weeks. Listen carefully to others and you will hear similar complaints along with their accompanying explanations. I agree with you that John Vincent's complaints now begin to sound absurd. Once you begin to do analyses of yourself and others, you will notice unusual nuances of behavior. Those who tell you their ills become unusually attentive to your reactions. Do you sympathize? Do you share similar ills and are you willing to trade stories? The John Vincents tell their stories with a twinge of embarrassment almost as if to say, "The illness or injury was my fault, but let's forget that for the moment." Am I reading into people's responses too much? Please observe yourself and others; judge for yourself.

Now let us look at John Vincent's specific complaints and see how we might interpret them. This is dangerous business to interpret for others and I make no claims to be right. I am just suggesting the avenues of inquiry that present themselves. Overall, the John Vincents tend to see the day as a series of threats from the external environment. Their physical health may be threatened by weather conditions, foods, pollens, lack of essential vitamins and minerals, electrolytes, improper warmups for exercise, breaks in routine, and the potential of a stressful day. All of these threats and their corresponding antidotes receive reinforcement from what we read in the print media and see on television. We are all assaulted by the possibilities of cancer, heart disease, AIDS, emphysema—the list goes on. In our culture, we are taught not to be passive in our responses, so for every disease we have the antidote suggested—broccoli and cauliflower, low-fat diets, social isolation, stop smoking. To prolong

157

existence, one must travel through a minefield. This is the reality as it is fed to us. As you might suspect, I have very mixed feelings about this information.

First, if we hear about antidotes or preventatives and totally ignore or defy them, we may be looking to catch a disease. We eat the fatty hamburger to clog our arteries and smoke the cigarettes to foul our lungs. Our use of the forbidden may be considered like a deliberate act to injure ourselves, such as stepping on a nail. Or, once we have the metaphor of fat and clogged arteries, our bodies use the metaphor to develop these conditions. Either way, once we have knowledge of the forbidden, the it may use these "external causes" to create disease. The illnesses we hear about also make contagion possible, another reason why I have mixed feelings about what I hear. Everyday we hear from others, read, or see the possibilities for dozens of diseases and injuries. Along with the antidotes go powerful suggestions as to what we could catch to bring sympathy to ourselves.

If I may anticipate your comments and criticisms, I am not reversing my former position about cause interna. First, I am suggesting that every disease we hear about suggests a possibility. Every antidote suggests to us a way of avoiding or catching a disease whether or not the antidote has any validity. The it may catch the cold it wants because the individual has conveniently forgotten his or her vitamin C.

To this point you probably have no quarrel with me. What about data that show a relationship between diet and heart disease, smoking and cancer? Only some of this data can be explained away by my previous example. In one sense, this data support my contention that we deliberately make ourselves ill. I spoke long distance to a friend last night and briefly mentioned my thesis. He said, "I sure know we are self-destructive. I must want to get ill or die for I smoke and overeat." Many ignore the advice they get and continue with their habits. Either through metaphor, actual damage to the body, or both, the use of the forbidden may contribute to disease. Perhaps you may call it a hedge, but I still am careful of what I eat.

The most serious objection you might have is, if there is evidence of environmental cause, why do you begin with cause interna? In the past letters I believe I answered that. We catch diseases and take on illnesses. The environment may be slightly dangerous to us, but we often contribute to illnesses by grabbing at the dangers. If there are now identified dangers like foods, pesticides, and perhaps many unknowns, how can we avoid illness? Each illness may have an internal and external cause. We help mightily when we create the cause interna. We can do our best to fend off the cause externa. As in the example of my friend Hank, we can choose to make ourselves the passive victims or choose not to.

Let us take a look at some of John Vincent's specific ills. He views himself in a titanic struggle with the environment. Onions will give him gas, the weather will make his postnasal drip worse, sugar will keep him awake, and running up the hill will injure his leg. He thinks of himself as a person of courage. I know, because for years I felt the same way. Consciously aware of the dangers, I fought off sickness and injury. This is what made accepting that I was the cause much more difficult. Let me suggest that what we often pick as conscious explanations greatly miss the mark. The party, not onions, will give him gas. Perhaps he does not want to see someone. The gas is an excuse to leave. There are studies now that show that if we believe ourselves to be allergic, just the thought or smell of the food may set off a reaction. The same spurious correlations may exist with the sugar, the hill, and the weather. We may have made those associations before with illness and injury, and they recur to bring symptoms. It has been my own experience and the experience of those I have taught that such spurious correlations, and the fact that they can sometimes become prophesies fulfilled, can be overcome.

Environmental, external causes can now become primary causes once associated with a disease. We mysteriously get gas at parties. Now we can conjure up gas by eating onions and postnasal drip by observing weather changes. These secondary causes as well as the primary causes can be overcome by understanding our role in the creation of illness and injury. What clever beings we are and how suggestible. If we can take pills and use metaphors as placebos, think how crafty we can be to use spurious correlations, fear of contagion, and suggestions of others to create disease and injury. How clever we are.

I hope I have answered your objections to my ideas. Before I conclude this letter I must anticipate—always a dangerous game—what may be at base your strongest resistance to these ideas. I want to convince you that I am right. Perhaps I am selfless in trying to help others to relieve their burdens, but you are too smart to fall for that. In some way I want your sympathies, your approval. "Dad," you might say, "you're a genius, right, saved my life, and so forth." Scott, you are correct in sniffing those motives out, for they are there in all of us when we speak or write. Critics are correct in suggesting that the self-sufficient, autonomous existentialist makes sure he has literary executors. It is a hedge to insure future generation sympathizers over and against the possibility of annihilation.

What makes this all so paradoxical is that by presenting ourselves in the past as ill, we have been able to gather up the sympathy of others. Think of the difficult reversal here that a father and son would have to make. In accepting my ideas, you would be expressing praise and admiration. At the same time, you would be giving up the basis for eliciting sympathy from me. Illness would become your problem and not my cause for concern. This is something that is very difficult to let go of. After all, perhaps my concern about you, as addressed in these letters, would fall off. The hero, the healthy, receives less attention.

As long as you show an interest in my theories but do not accept them, you have got me. Up to this point, I have enjoyed our little duel. Further efforts to convince you would be redundant and not solve the major problem, whether we look at it as a problem of sympathy or power, or simply that the facts show you are right and I am wrong. Now you can see why I try to teach others to analyze themselves and do not want to help them work out the analyses; I am a teacher, not an analyst. To be well means to give up one's relationship with an analyst. It is almost too much to ask.

So, I leave you alone with Groddeck, Augie, and future thoughts on the subject. In future letters I will try to avoid the subject.

Love,

Dad

Letters to B. J.

Dear B. J.,

It is so good to hear from you again. Now that you have caught up with me and read *Groddeck* and some of my early essays, I am eager to push on and tell you of some ideas that have occurred to me during our hiatus. First, let me comment on the analyses you did on yourself and offer my congratulations. I guess the breakthrough for you was your water-ski trip. Your brother, as I remember, had urged you for years to try waterskiing, and you always managed to turn him down. Perhaps in our correspondence, you could investigate and find out why you had this fear. Nonetheless, your it found a clever way out this time. You had reluctantly decided to go waterskiing, and your ankle began to hurt on the way to the lake. At the insistence of your brother (I wonder why getting you to ski was so important to him), you continued to the lake. The pain peaked when you got there and served as an excuse to go home. Very interesting that all the pain was gone by the time you got home again. Next time you are asked to go, if you have not gotten over your reluctance to water-ski, you will refuse.

Yes, you are the first person I am aware of who got the measles three times. Each time it was before you went to a dance in high school. You are aware, of course, that Groddeck often found that teenagers developed skin eruptions before such events. Your measles really insured you would stay home from the prom.

I single out these examples of yours because they show that you have seen the process work in illness and injury and can apply the analysis to current as well as past events. Most ingenious is your analysis of your bladder infections. Your husband's death caused you a great deal of guilt as you describe it. You need not be so harsh on yourself, but that is another matter. Your subsequent marriage seemed to go smoothly except for the infection which made you hold back on intercourse. It is a good thing you discovered that you withheld sex out of fear of hurting your late husband's feelings. Lucky, too, that understanding this principle was enough to make the infection disappear. This example was excellent for it showed not only that you could understand the process but also that you could bring on changes yourself.

Your waterskiing example reminds me that once we understand the principles, we can be in the business of prevention as well as cure. I can avoid headaches if I do not watch TV; waterskiing can be hazardous to your health. I follow the Denver Broncos, as you know. Invariably, as a player is about to lose his starting position or suffer some other loss of status, he gets hurt. The coaches could help prevent this by making a special effort to encourage those players about to be demoted. A coach has to fight giving all his attention to current favorites. If I were experimentally inclined, I would study who was having good and bad games. Then I would correlate this with injury. Sure there are two or more involved in these accidents, but how careful are we to prevent injury; how well do we protect ourselves?

One of the ideas I have been toying with lately is that "everything works." Since the work of Hans J. Eysenck in England and Carl Rogers in the United States, people have been trying to prove that therapies bring change. Most of the results are mixed, and one study almost cynically shows that one-third improve, one-third stay the same, and one-third get worse. The debates are endless and fraught with methodological problems, for what are health and illness? With organic illnesses, we have the same types of problems in measuring success. Rollo May has convictions that alleviation of psychological traumas can cure some illnesses. Barbara Brown has been doing excellent work with biofeedback. Others work with guided imagery. Faith healers are ever present with their claims. And followers of Hans Selye have gone farthest with empirical data showing the relationship between life crises and illness. Both in England and the United States, over one hundred forty therapies are practiced. Overall, the results are mixed.

I can chalk up the mixed results to methodological problems by our experimentally minded brothers and sisters. What are health and illness? Do we have enough comparable cases? Are some researchers careless or dishonest? Do researchers look for correlation only, or do they go in with research hypotheses? All these work to give us mixed results. Look at any major issue in the social sciences; the more the evidence piles up, the more confusing the results are. This is the "law of mixed results."

I know, given this skepticism, I could just as well say nothing works as well as everything works. My own observations and readings allow me to see positive results from lots of different approaches. Success is often dependent on the skill of the worker applying his or her therapy. As well, success depends even more, I am convinced, on the willingness of the patient's it. Groddeck felt that by and large we cure ourselves and I agree. I have instructed many people in my methods, and success seems only marginally related to my performance. I still hold that everything works, but certainly not for all people. Someone could go from my class, remember nothing, and after many other therapies, be "cured" by a faith healer. In psychoanalytic circles, it is well known that certain therapists have success with certain types of clients. Referrals are often made on this basis.

As I have mentioned before, the family therapists have made great strides in explaining success or lack of it, if we use their concept of a "presenting problem." If a family comes to a therapist for help, the therapist should begin with the problem as conceived by the family. When I teach my philosophy and other alternatives, ideas succeed if people view their lives in the same way. I do not teach to cure illness, but to speak of alternative modes of living well, from Plato's *Republic* and More's *Utopia* to Groddeck's skeptical vitalism. I have not found the way nor if I do find the way, am I about to use it to coerce others to virtue. I am happy in my role of disseminating Groddeck's ideas and my own.

So I have made the tenuously substantiated statement that everything works and shown why everything fails as well. Yet, B. J., the fact that everything works substantiates the claims that Groddeck and I make that our philosophical position and psychological position are sound. A neat trick if I can put it past you.

If we look at the history of the treatment of disease, one fact comes easily to mind. Healers have always used striking metaphors in their diagnoses and treatments. Today we have in the field of mental illness the medical model where symptoms are clustered and labeled as diseases. The exotic names of diseases with their self-contained and isolatable symptoms seem to be prime targets for some weapon: a pill, a scalpel, a revelation—be it psychoanalytic or religious—which could exorcise the symptoms. Boils may be lanced, nerves be tranquilized with pills, demons be exorcised, and viruses and bacteria be killed. If we go back to Greek times, we see how prominent was the metaphor. For Hippocrates, man was warmest the first day of his existence and coldest the last. This heat emanated from the heart; it was the flame that fired his existence. Poets still use the metaphor of the flame.

The theory of humors which dominated medicine for so long is rich with metaphors. Health or temperance exists when there is the proper mixture of humors. There was blood, phlegm, yellow bile, and black bile. Treatment too used metaphor. Never change the diet drastically for the humors might fly even more out of kilter. Boiling water had excellent properties; sweet wine was too heavy. Do not feed or fuel a fever. The overall metaphor for the Greeks was moderation, which applied to health as well as politics. Interestingly enough, the temperance metaphor is once again in vogue where doctors are suggesting that maintaining a constant weight is most important for health.

I know I may be running on as if I am lecturing, but see if you draw the same conclusions from the use of metaphor as I do. In the eighteenth century, metaphors of fluids and mechanics took over. There was a belief that anger, joy, and lust were caused by excessive tension in the nervous fibers or excessive activity of the body fluids. In contrast, fear, depression, and ennui, even stupidity, were caused by the opposites: weak brain marrow and nervous fibers or sluggish fluids. Cures were designed to reach a mean. We have the idea of humors, fluids, and fibers following us into the nineteenth century.

The cures are interesting from the standpoint of metaphor as well. In 1662, Moritz Hoffman suggested a complete transfusion for melancholics to get rid of the bad blood. Bitter coffee was thought to get rid of thickened humors of an overweight person. Soapy fruits like cherries and strawberries could dissolve humors and bad fluids. Water, if hot, could increase passion or, if cool, could decrease passion. Cold water immersion could shock someone back to "reality." Whole therapies were devised around cures that could open or close pores: exercise could cleanse bodies of impurities; baths could open pores; food could clean out poisons.

Remember now that I am speaking of the metaphor in medicine, not a history of archaic practices. I began with the current illness metaphor and the metaphor associated with cures. We have medicines that relax muscles, kill germs fast, coat stomach linings, contain double pain-reliever, and absorb gas; I could go on and on. You might say these are over-the-counter medicines, but even your doctor will tell you in metaphors what a prescription medicine will do for you.

Now you can see why everything works. Even those ancient cures, in which the metaphors to describe the body were only roughly descriptive of actual processes, allowed people to visualize disease before healing occurred. What is necessary is belief in the metaphor. This is why some doctors are more effective than others. Faith healers get their clients to visualize God as the agency of cure; an over-the-counter medicine gets the patient to see a coating on his or her stomach. This is why medicine was always somewhat effective even though "cures" may today be found to have no medicinal properties. The doctor or healer gives to the patient sympathy, comfort, and a credible metaphor, and shows obvious pleasure at improvement. The patient must do the rest: want a cure, accept the metaphor, and get well. Perhaps this idea is best understood by the people working with biofeedback and guided imagery.

Now I hope you can see why I say that everything works. Next I need to show you, although you have probably guessed, why I stick to my methods. Obviously, my explanation of cure lies with the idea of one person speaking in symbols to another person's it. These beans have a coppery taste, and if you eat them, you will get a sour stomach. Take this medicine, and your stomach will be coated. The metaphor suggests an avenue for cure, and the person delivering the metaphor can provide the motivation. On the way back from the lake, perhaps your brother said that your swelled ankle would take a week to go down by itself, but only a few days if you applied ice to reduce the swelling or stayed off it so as not to aggravate the sore tendons. Think back to your trip to the lake and see if anyone suggested an appropriate recovery.

Groddeck not only enhances his theory with the idea of symbol and metaphor but also goes on to show why we sometimes accept metaphors and at other times reject them. We are better off if we can understand our own motivations. Why do we accept some cures and reject others? The theory Groddeck and I share describes the dynamics behind the illness and the cure as well as the importance of the relationship between the deliverer of the metaphor and his or her interaction with the recipient. Our theory explains why "everything works."

Keep well,

Augie

Jog to get your blood circulating in the morning.
Brush your hair vigorously to strengthen the roots.
Eat six to eight times a day to keep your stomach slightly full and active.

These can spur you on to health, but noncompliance could bring on a guilt and illness. So—

Wake up slowly so as not to jolt your system; do not jog.
Gently brush your hair or it will irritate the roots.
Eat three hearty meals a day.

As you see, the practice of medicine is very tricky.

Dear B. J.,

The analyses you did on yourself are quite interesting and show you have grasped the basic principles. That alone should be enough to show you why I prefer that people learn the techniques rather than asking me to do formal analysis with them. But you ask interesting questions: "Why write a philosophy? Why not practice as a therapist?" I will not formally dodge the answer. The reason the question is so difficult is that my reasons may be tricks of my it. In brief, I prefer not to be a therapist, although others might successfully practice as Groddeckian analysts. Let me go into a few of the professional reasons why I do not practice and then consider the advantages of practicing on one's self.

As you know, I do not have the formal credentials of the analyst. In our society, this stops few people from finding an institutional base from which to operate. I could go into private consultation with my wife. In other words, obstacles to a private practice are not insurmountable. Therefore, I feel the major reasons I do not practice lie elsewhere.

I am not tempted to do more than show others how to do analyses. Perhaps one of the reasons for my reluctance is that I am not interested in such work. Philip Roth makes the distinction between therapy and analysis. The former is the reassurances given, the games of sympathy and repetition that are played with patients. I know that a therapist can cut these to a minimum. A debate rages right now in psychoanalysis between practitioners who will make sympathetic remarks to those whom they treat (for example, acknowledge with sorrow the death of a loved one) and others who feel this sympathy is an intervention that may interfere with analysis. Perhaps the client was not sorry the person died and would feel guilty about the analyst's sympathy. In either school of thought, much time is spent on games with patients, even if reassurance is not the goal. To some, all of this is fascinating, but personally I do not have the patience. Analysis, learning something new about the patient and his or her world is interesting, but too time consuming for me. In my early Groddeckian phase, I can tell you I spent much time on these enterprises. Now I leave therapy to others.

If these are personal motives, I would like to feel that through awareness I have settled this question of educating others or giving therapy, although I know my it may be playing tricks on me. Groddeck went from a strategy of authoritative commands that he learned from Schweninger to a position of non-judgmental intervention. According to reports of patients as well as from his own letters, we learn he rarely intervened. In this way, he was much closer to contemporaries of mine such as the late Carl Rogers than to the early analysts. For Groddeck, the person's it would decide to make the organism well.

Karen Horney wrote a marvelous book about the individual doing self-analysis. If you read her volume, it will satisfy many of the questions I do not answer. What is interesting to note is her defensiveness about self-analysis and the necessity of describing it as second best to seeking professional help. This clearly reflects the attitude of most analysts: the doctor should be in charge and professional training is necessary.

I feel that the necessary progression is teaching others to analyze themselves. With little more than the Delphic injunction to know themselves, Freud and Groddeck showed that self-analysis, or what I would rather call the search for life through awareness, could be accomplished. For me, the search for life through awareness was a lot easier, for I had the advice of Freud, Groddeck, Horney, and many others. Rather than looking at self-inquiry as a necessary burden, I look at it as a virtue.

If you try to heighten your own awareness, you manage to retain your own freedom. In one important way you are not playing on the sympathies of another when you are examining your own life. You are not confirming the hypotheses of another or rejecting them when you do your own analyses. I know that the best of analysts can do a pretty good job at hiding their own hypotheses, but the patient is also observer and, even under a minimum of intervention by the analyst, can discern the analyst's views. There is no concern about trying to please or anger the analyst when you examine your own life.

To use psychoanalytic terms, transference as well as counter-transference takes place in analyses. These processes get in the way of strengthening your own awareness. You begin responding to the person who faces you. Part of the genius of Freud was to use the setback of transference as a way to find out more about the patient. In transference, the patient begins to act towards the analyst in the same way that he or she behaves towards others in the present, as well as when the patient was younger. If the directive analyst could explain transference to the patient or if the nondirective analyst could get the patient to see transference for what it is, much would be accomplished in analysis. From being a drawback to the analysis of another person, transference becomes a virtue. Transference becomes a major therapeutic tool. Debates still rage about this technique: degrees of intrusiveness necessary, degrees of intimacy with patient, termination of therapy, and many others. Transference is a lot of things—useful, tricky, controversial. If I chose to be an analyst, no doubt I would have to find good use for it as a therapeutic tool. (With self analysis, you keep free of the transference and retain your own freedom.) As I hope to show you, you still have use for the idea but do not have to worry about it in therapy. In terms a friend of mine uses, you need only to speak to yourself about yourself. That is fraught with more than enough pitfalls.

The search for life through awareness is freedom in more than one way. You search when you want, you do it for free, and most importantly, cure is not the only goal. In therapy, you may determine what the problems are to be dealt with, but concerns of time and money as well as pace and obligation come up. These may seem trivial, but they are not. A good analyst may set you at ease with your explorations, but limits will always be imposed. The best of analysts will keep them to a minimum.

I am only speaking for myself, B. J. To others, freedom may not loom as important. They may want to examine life through a cooperative effort. Good luck to them. My only goal is to show that the search for life through awareness can be done alone—and one need not apologize for doing so. What I am arguing for is an examined life, one in which we are responsible for what we find and for the actions based on these findings. Reading Freud, Groddeck, Horney, and others may be very helpful in suggesting how to proceed, and I would not pretend to go at it alone. We need all the help we can get. Nor would I advise you or anyone else to stay away from analysts. They can be the best teachers. All I ask is that you keep in mind your own freedom and take ultimate responsibility for your being. This can be difficult to retain in a long-standing relationship with another. Existential psychotherapists are perhaps most acutely aware of this problem. But even the best of them still must convince those they comfort that the ultimate goal is to be free. So you see, B. J., I am not hardheaded on the subject. Others with inclinations similar to mine may be doing useful therapy and teaching patients to know themselves and act for themselves.

Before I mention some potential drawbacks of self-inquiry, I will set forth some of its strengths. Of prime importance when you do self-analysis is to remember there is no need for commitment to a set of outcomes or possibilities. In the presence of an analyst, you would be asked to find, and probably would find, a curse in your past, which would take on some degree of importance. All this of course is based on positive transference taking place. Free of an analyst, however, you may develop your own structures and methods. When not in the presence of authority, you are in a stronger position to innovate. By increasing awareness of your own life, you are involved in an enterprise broader than the one defined by the analyst (obvious exceptions) and feel bathed in great luxury. Knowing yourself is merely a part of a field of concerns you might have about life and the world.

In my next letter I will tell you of some of the pitfalls of exploring life and expanding your awareness. You are probably already aware of many pitfalls since you expressed your reservations about self-analysis. After that, I will suggest some of the techniques you can use in expanding awareness. I will give you this instruction not because you need it, but because it will bolster your confidence.

Augie

———————— ❦ ————————

Dear B. J.,

As I promised, I will speak of some of the problems of self-inquiry. Given my belief in self-analysis, I will deliver the criticisms without great zeal or enthusiasm. There are too many benefits to self-analysis: the potential for freedom in inquiry; sidestepping an analyst who could potentially be the target for sympathy; my modest success along with that of Freud and Groddeck, among others, who have successfully analyzed themselves.

The most serious problem may be that you begin to report your successes and failures in self-analysis to others. If you do not take care, this person may become the object of transference. Another person's approval of your explanations, his or her questioning of your enterprise, could greatly influence what you find, just as if you were doing the analysis with this individual as your analyst. If this reporting to another occurs, you must analyze this transference and, just as the psychoanalyst does, let it help you with your inquiry. Even if you tell no one about the analysis, be careful that you do not have a potential audience in mind. The person does not have to be present to be thought of as a recipient of certain thoughts or behaviors. At some later date, I will elaborate, but for now, I will warn you that we usually have an audience in mind for our thoughts and actions.

Along the same lines, those we read in order to learn how to analyze ourselves may create a situation of transference for us. Groddeck bears a strong resemblance to an uncle of mine, and as I read his works, I had to fight a tranference. As I re-read Freud, I fought an anger (judge not) that I felt toward him because he did not listen carefully to Groddeck's ideas. Beware my letters and writings in the same way.

Other criticisms of self-inquiry come to mind all too easily: some people are not in a position to help themselves; analysts could spread the gospel more quickly and help more people; in general, telling people to help themselves through increasing their own awareness is not a populist approach to the problem. These problems are probably the ones that vex you the most. Let me answer you here.

I could begin and end my statement by saying that I am a philosopher who has discovered for himself ideas about truth and being that are sufficient in themselves. The results have been published and there is no more to it. Almost every writer, however, including me, becomes a "political" philosopher in musing about how his or her ideas will be disseminated and received. If we argue that our writings are for ourselves alone, that we have no other audience, then we protest too much. Groddeck, for example, continually writes that he wants no followers for they weigh him down, that he is a doctor out of habit and helping people is incidental, that he has no need for recognition. Groddeck protests too much. His letters to Freud implore the latter to take account of his views and respect his ideas. Groddeck shows great anger and disappointment at different times in his correspondence. He displays desperation in wanting his books published and anxiety over Otto Rank's editorial hand on his *Book of the It*. In other words, even Groddeck was concerned with the politics of his ideas, from his initial disappointment that Freud, not he, was the first to publish their explorations on the unconscious to his disappointment that Freud would not come to Baden-Baden to be cured of cancer.

I agree with Groddeck on his point that we do not necessarily want to help others for altruistic reasons; we may be trying to prove to our fathers that we are competent, fear being thought of as selfish, or have many reasons for wanting to help/dominate others. Whatever the reason, whether pure altruism or a Hobbesian need for domination, we cannot, like Groddeck, deny the politics of our ideas. I write to you and for others because I want you and others to understand my ideas, try the same processes, and have the same results. My reasons may in fact be sweet or ugly. The discipline comes in allowing others the freedom to accept my ideas or to reject them . Before I sound too altruistic, I must admit that allowing others their freedom may be the best way to get them to utilize my ideas. I may derive more satisfaction from persuasion than domination.

So you see, B. J., the question of why I propose self-inquiry, of expanding awareness—done without intervention—is not a simple one. I would love to conclude that my love for freedom turned into a Kantian imperative is all there is to my proposals. Groddeck has allowed me to extend these freedoms even further. At the same time, Groddeck forces me to consider my underlying motives for acting. I cannot deny that I wish others would freely choose *my* ideas.

Your suggestion to include these letters in a volume of collected readings is a good one. Groddeck's protest about putting his ideas in print does not ring true. Nobody had to twist his arm. What I intend to do is convince others of my philosophy. I discipline myself to respect the freedom of others, but for more devious reasons known by my it, I will continue to argue for self-analysis.

To your freedom,

Augie

Dear B. J.,

You spotted something very interesting in my ideas that I was unaware of. I espouse freedom through awareness, but although I can try to command another through awareness, the it of the other may not receive my message in the way intended. I can learn, as Milton Erickson and Groddeck did, to communicate to the it of another, but interpretation of my message ultimately depends on the receiver.

Let me give you an example of how I tried to enhance another's freedom by coercing him through awareness to my views and how his it balked at the message. You know my friend Steve and how I have told him about my ideas since their inception. I never twisted his arm, but I refined my arguments on him. He was my *ficelle* in this drama. The more I wanted his approval (conversion), the more he resisted. I will not go into the transferences set up, but they made the talks difficult. He kept returning to disprove my theory. The other day he came in and told me that through guided imagery he had cured a headache. Reading the work of others, he had found a way to do what I had done through Groddeck. I was thrilled. He had found the perfect way to maintain his freedom while remaining in contact with me.

The Strangelove in me came out in the situation. Not content to leave Steve with the illusion of freedom, I pointed out that I had originally suggested that organic illnesses could be cured by reference to mental processes. Furthermore, I told him how "everything works" to effect a cure. In addition, I reminded him how Groddeck and I could explain and relativize the views of those who use guided imagery (the metaphor) to cure. Under the kindly guise of explaining why it worked, I reminded him of his indebtedness to his teacher. My attempt to extend freedom to myself and others broke down. Looking back, I am excited by what happened despite my slight transgression. He freely

179

interpreted my teaching and worked out a solution to his problems on his own. He chose to listen because illness plagued him. Guided imagery fit in with his use of religion and imagination in solving problems. As I continue to analyze what happened, I must thank you, B. J., for reminding me that giving others their freedom revolves on the issue of how people are selective in what they hear. Compliance would only be on the surface, on the level of awareness.

At this juncture I know you want me to give an idea of methods I use to increase my awareness. The key to method is the linkage between our it and illness. Access can be gained in many ways. I will show you what some means of access are. Others have been covered in earlier letters. First, I want to give you an illustration of something that is just occurring and illustrates how many ways we gain access. Beware, however, the dangers of a manual on methods is that it can stifle your own imagination.

Tuesday (today is Thursday) following my afternoon class, I ran. My running partner said he felt great, and I returned that I felt lousy. I was experiencing sharp pains in various parts of my stomach, some resembling the symptoms of appendicitis. Since Monday night they had come intermittently. I recall this now, but I had paid scant attention to the pains; they were not severe. As you can see, I am not forever taking my pulse. I had given no time to analyzing the pain because I was busy.

Last night I had a dream. In the dream I was at a convention and tried to give a paper. I was drowned out. (Perhaps my concern about the politics of writing.) At one point I was given a chance to speak, but a good friend of mine sat on my stomach and I could not speak loudly enough to tell him I had to take a train. I managed to jump on the train with another friend at the last minute and found out that the train would stop to view architectural sights along the way. We sat next to the tour director and did not have the courage to tell him to keep going on and not stop at the sights.

I woke up from this dream and, as I do on such occasions, went into the den and meditated on it. I try not to open my eyes on the way downstairs in order to "keep" the dream. (A neat trick stumbling down the stairs over shoes and clothing.) This saves me many efforts of recall. My way of analyzing the dream is to let my mind free as I slowly do stretching exercises. I am not proposing the method to you, but simply explaining to show you how idiosyncratic we can be.

My thoughts kept drifting from the dream to other ideas. I became aware of a rumination I had been having over the past few days. My mind repeatedly switched from dream to rumination; both were variants of the same thing. In the class that meets just before I jog on Tuesdays, a student who speaks labored English, but with a great deal of zeal, ranted to the class about Jews, bankers, and exploiters. Last night, a colleague, in the course of a conversation, compared my behavior to a colleague of mine who was also Jewish. Was there the insinuation that this was "typical" behavior? Other matters of this sort made up the rumination including Jacobo Timerman's stance that one should never be ashamed of being a Jew. For months I have been ruminating over his ideas. Also, I thought of my conversation yesterday with a colleague who had a student defiantly put his legs up on the seat in a large lecture class. I gave him advice on how to handle the situation.

These themes interlaced in the dream. What I wanted to do in the dream was to get up in the fashion of Timerman and announce that I was Jewish. The incident of the girl ranting in class had brought up a long-standing problem with me. As you know, people never identify me as a Jew. As a consequence, I hear remarks not intended for a Jew's ears. People speak of "jewing" others down. On a train back to college, I met a person I had played against in high school basketball. He said that he was pleased to beat Hewlett, a school in our conference, for they were a bunch of Jews. Most recently, a fireman in a conversation mentioned something I had never heard, "Jewish lightning." This is where someone intentionally sets a fire to collect insurance.

My problem is always how to respond. In the last case, a glare brought a mumbled apology to the effect that he did not know why such a statement was made. However, most of the time I have felt ineffectual in these situations. In the dream provoked by the class incident, this friend was sitting on me. He is one I have long suspected had anti-Semitic feelings even though we are friends. I could not tell him to get off me. My companion on the train, as helpless as I to tell the conductor (bigot) to change his ways, was my friend whom I had advised to get tough with his misbehaving student (a projection on my part), and he seemed as powerless as I.

Through a dream I found the rumination, but I had not yet linked it to illness. The wish was to express myself as a Jew and not to shrink from embarrassment for myself or the other person. I realized that I had to solve this problem and to say in class today that I am a Jew. The problem was not the inchoate woman's but mine. The solution I reached after searching for various alternatives is as follows: I am teaching political theory in this course, and last period I asked all of the students to write a sentence that expressed some important idea they have or some important influence on them. In the next class, I will deal with my "idea" first. My idea is that early experiences influence our political philosophy—no great shakes I admit, simply the standard Freud-Lasswell formula. My illustration will be how as a child I was speaking to a friend in a candy story and said I would like to be president of the United States someday. The store owner, one of little stature both in the community and among the kids, said, "A Jew can never be president." I was shocked, outraged. What were my limits? Perhaps it is no coincidence that I became a political scientist, have existential leanings, and will not let anyone else determine my limits. In class today, I will recount this story from my childhood. As a result, the student will have the choice of continuing in my class or withdrawing from it. I will tell the story without directly embarrassing her and, more importantly, I will speak with candor.

After I made this decision, I noticed that my pains had disappeared. This bout with stomach pains was a reproof of my silence at the candy store and with my student. The pains returned later when I thought of the possibility that she might not be in class but they are gone now because I am convinced I will go through with my plan whenever she returns to class.

So you see, we can get to the it in various ways. We can create our own methods. If we just look for the link between illness and the it, we may cure ourselves many times over. A look at this linkage may show how dealing with problems in the past may have often cured ills. If I had dealt with this student without making the linkage between illness and candor, I would have been cured anyway. (My argument still favors seeking awareness in this situation, because now I will understand the problem.) And this remains my argument with those who use other cures. You can always fire "bullets" through guided imagery to kill a disease, but if you follow my methods—here I go again—you will know more about yourself and prevent recurrence.

In the above explanation, see an example of the curse/blessing that led to my existentialism, the present rumination, and the action to effect the cure. What remains is to explain the pains of appendicitis. I think of the appendix and I think of vestigial organ and I think of Judaism for my life. If someone is accusatory of Jews, my it prepares my appendix for removal. Easier to remove the vestigial organ than to admit the Jew is in me.

Next time I will speak more of method.

Augie

A *Jew* with an appendix

Dear B. J.,

I did leave you hanging on the outcome of the encounter with my opinionated student. The reason I wrote as if the incident were finished is that I was definite in my plans and was convinced as to how I would carry it through. I followed through in the precise manner I described. The student sat there frozen as I spoke, betraying no particular feelings. Now it is her choice as to whether or not she returns to the class. The whole class was directed at her, but general enough to be of interest to others. I never, of course, mentioned her or said anything that would single her out to the others.

As I sat down to write to you about method, a student of mine came in to talk to me about Groddeck's *Book of the It* which she had started to read. I have known her for over a year, and when she expressed curiosity about my work, I introduced her to Groddeck with the proper warnings. What I propose to do is relate the conversation I had with her to show you how I teach someone to do analysis.

Barb was familiar with my ideas and had begun to observe the behavior of others with respect to illness. She had tried to analyze her own illnesses, but without much success. Her pressing complaint was, How do you know something is true? I explained to her about how all associations are true. Using Freud's concept of overdetermination, I explained that she may have several explanations for the same circumstance. When you make all these associations, you will be affected emotionally by some more than others. Do not think strong emotion is always a revelation. Follow Leslie Farber's injunction to allow the thoughts to settle and look again—reexamine your analysis.

My conversation with Barb began when she told me she had been reading Groddeck's chapter four while eating dinner and she suddenly lost her appetite. Always look for *specificity* in circumstances that surround the onset of an illness. Look for even the most minute details. She was reading a book. She was reading chapter four. She was reading about pregnancy and the voluptuous feelings of giving birth. Groddeck also mentioned constipation in that chapter.

I am showing her how to do analysis and from now on she will do it herself. An hour is enough to begin to teach someone who has access to my works, Freud's, or Groddeck's. I asked her what the consequences were of reading this section and losing her appetite. I explained that I could only guess for her, but an answer could take several forms: lack of appetite could cause her to leave the table and put down the book which was disturbing her; lack of appetite could cause her to spend less money this month; etc. As you will see later, Barb's explanation was far more interesting. At this point in our conversation, the best she could come up with was that talking about constipation could make one lose one's appetite. "Doesn't everyone react this way?" she asked. I explained that when people first respond to such questions they often come up with mundane answers that seem to be shared by everyone. The first associations they make are socially acceptable ones. I quickly commented that neither I nor my friends would be bothered by the association of constipation and childbirth. Certainly that association would not decrease our appetites.

I must digress and tell you I do this pedantic instruction explicitly to allow the person to work through alone the next set of problems she or he faces. At this point, I became aware that even though Barb had read about it-talk, she needed to see a demonstration. I told her that one of the many threads I was following in analyzing myself was the question of why I got headaches when I watched TV. My associations had led me to see myself as a child with a wooden hammer pounding cylindrical blocks down into their slots. When they were down, I turned the apparatus over and pounded them down again. This device was a distraction for me then, as the TV is now. I also remember that my mother was in the next room and I did not want to hear something that was going on. Barb interrupted and asked, "Do your parents fight?" I said that like all parents they argued. She had made a good guess. (Now is a good time to show you the pitfalls of intruding on someone else's analysis. As I think about this picture I have of the above events, it was my mother and someone other than my father arguing. Barb had talked me into seeing my parents as the antagonists.)

I said to Barb that free association cannot be too intentional and we cannot worry where we end up. I am convinced that as we do our it-talk, we eventually work our way back to our rumination. I began associating out loud and said the first thing I thought about was the hammer. The hammer made me think of tongs which made me think of the Chinese which made me think of chow mein. From there I recalled going to a Chinese restaurant that belonged to a man who was taught English by my uncle. I remembered he would treat us like royalty and then charge the going rate. Praise and appreciation for my uncle and his family were verbal, and not translated into a discount. We ate and paid royally. Then, as I told Barb, I remembered saying a derogatory set of words that would demean one who was Chinese. My father scolded me, and I was thoroughly ashamed and embarrassed.

The above demonstration of it-talk was meant to show Barb the range of ideas and the freedom permitted and to encourage her to loosen up and try the method. Ultimately I instruct the student as to how it-talk leads to insight.

Barb asked me if you always get back to the problem you started with, and I said yes if you do it-talk enough. I did not provide her with an example at the time. Let me now tell you what occurs as I write these lines, to show you (unfortunately I was not able to show Barb at the time) how our associations come full circle back to a rumination. It also shows how you can pick up on prior it-talk and continue associations.

When I used the derogatory terms, I was trying to help my father who had shown displeasure in the restaurant at such treatment by the proprietor. More importantly, my mother was angry at my father's inaction; she felt he should have demanded a cheaper tab. Thinking I would straighten things out between them by insulting the proprietor, I blurted out, "Chinky, Chinky, chow mein!" Instead of being pleased with my effort, my father angrily told me to mind my own business.

I saw a relationship between the incident at the Chinese restaurant, my mother's arguing with a stranger while I pounded cylinders, and the headaches I get while watching TV. At the restaurant I tried in a peculiar way to assuage my mother's anger by standing in for my father, but I was reprimanded for my attempt. So, when my mother was arguing with someone in the next room, I chose not to help her. To block out the anger I was sure she felt at my inaction, I vigorously pounded cylinders into my toy. In my adult life, the TV has replaced my childhood hammer and cylinders; both have served as diversions to block out unpleasantness. Therefore, when I watch TV, I recall my mother's anger at inaction—mine when she was arguing (or so I thought) and my father's at the restaurant. Invariably, I get a headache.

I go only a step further here, for my purpose is to show you how associations work and come full circle. My choice of the example for Barb (TV/toy) was related to a rumination of the day: the rumination that I want to see the Broncos play this weekend on TV. So you see, it all comes full circle. Why did I stop my analysis where I did? A resistance? Perhaps, but I need to get on with my story, and never fail, when I have my leisure, I will pick up the trail.

It-talk begins to loosen one up. Read Groddeck's it-talk—poetry—and you begin to relax and make associations. Read with leisure and do not be anxious to get back to the point of the story or poem. Barb would not have needed me at all if she had continued to muse about constipation, voluptuous births, and appetite. Suddenly she told me that she was adopted. She was going to go in a few weeks to her adoptive parents' home in Washington state, but more importantly, she was going to try to find her natural mother. Then she began musing that she envisions meeting her mother in a park. I asked her why. She said that a park is a beautiful setting and she wants her mother to see her at her best. Barb had begun to free associate in front of me. I tried to intervene only to instruct, but intervention brings no risk because a broken train of thought can always be picked up again.

As with Theodore Reik's listening with the third ear, I began to hear certain threads in Barb's conversation, not only today, but back over a period of visits. Sometimes the analyst can work best by picking up the threads and giving them to the student.

But I prefer to teach a student to listen to herself or himself with his or her own third ear. The learner then becomes aware of the rumination; in the discussion with Barb that followed, she made most of the connections. I pointed out a few of those I will specifically mention. She was about to leave school and was worried about what she should do for a career. She wanted to be in broadcast journalism, to practice law, or to teach political theory. I told her that she was capable of all three, but she must be careful about choosing the third option because she might be trying to please me. A short discussion followed when she said that she wanted to please her mother, her "real" mother.

I went on for a while about the legitimacy of ambivalent feelings towards people. She interrupted and seemed shocked. She said that she wanted to ask her mother what she should do for a career. Taking into consideration the general feelings of adopted individuals, I told her that whatever she found out about her mother she had already worked out in her head. I became a preacher and not a listener. I told her that whether her mother was intelligent or not (Barb's main concern), Barb could still do whatever she wanted. I told her I was giving her a blessing.

At this point, Barb spoke about being physically well this summer except for diarrhea which caused her to lose six pounds. Her weight was usually constant and she was surprised about this. Conversation continued on whether she would go through with seeing her mother and asking her mother what she thought about careers. I told her that if her mother did not give a satisfactory answer, I would counsel her on a career choice. Barb said, "Augie, I tried that and it didn't work." She hesitated, fidgeted a bit, and then answered that she was getting antsy and needed to leave. Her response was vehement. She had never before addressed me as Augie; I decided I had better ask her about what had just happened. I began with a Groddeck-like question: "What are the consequences of fidgeting?" "Because I am uncomfortable, I would have to leave," she answered. "Why do you want to leave? Because I am trying to dissuade you from looking for your mother?" I guessed. "Yes, damn it," was her response. She visibly relaxed, and I explained to her that I just wanted to assure her that I would be here after her visit to her mother, no matter what she found, and that she was a capable person. We relaxed and continued our conversation.

Again like a bolt she sat upright and said, "Now I know why I don't want to eat anymore. I want to be very presentable to my mother. All I was told about her was that she was slim and blonde." From this point Barb rapidly began making association after association. I will only recount some of them. She said, "My diarrhea was a way to lose weight. Just last week I began to swim every day." A whole range of activities that seemed to have no common origin were now related. Every person's ruminations are a novel or at least a short story wanting to be found. From Barb's first utterance to me today about Groddeck, voluptuous birth, and loss of appetite to her last thoughts with me today, she was expressing, unknown to herself, her rumination. Remember a person's (including your own) first and last remark to another, and you will often identify a rumination.

At this point, Barb looked very sheepish and said that something else was on her mind. She has known a graduate student casually for three years. Now he is out in Seattle and she has made plans to meet him. At this juncture, Barb said, "Of course, it is related! He is the perfect mate. I want to introduce him to my real mother."

The conversation took another turn when Barb said that her adoptive father always asks her to clean her plate; not doing so is a bit of a rebellion. (I did not follow this up, but a crude guess is that she is torn between her real and adoptive parents; to not eat is to get in shape for her real mother.) Until reading Groddeck, she rarely stopped eating before cleaning her plate. All this was clarified when I asked her why she now thinks she did not eat when she read Groddeck. She said that she had always admired her real mother for going through with her birth and not having an abortion. The voluptuous experience of birth removes some of the altruism in the mother's act of giving birth. Barb wanted to be like her mother (thin) and hoped that her mother would be as Barb had envisioned her.

We spoke for a while about what she had learned from the analysis. She realized she would have to listen with a third ear and continue thinking about the various threads she would have to follow. I congratulated her for now understanding Groddeck.

She interrupted me (probably embarrassed by my needless flattery) and said that she had put off seeing her real mother. She paid this month's rent on her apartment. She called her father and got him to agree (which was easy, for he dislikes waste) to her staying on until the end of the month since she had already paid for the apartment. I told her that I was not cursing her, but that she should analyze any sickness she might get in anticipation of her trip to Seattle.

Shooting myself in the foot by going on a mite too long, I told her to judge not and fear not the results of analysis, and gave her sundry other hints. She did not take umbrage, and in the Groddeckian way, I saw our conversation as a success.

So you see, B. J., this is how I teach people to do analysis. A little reading, a little on-site instruction. I will see Barb before she leaves, and I am sure she will have a few more questions. Once she has done an analysis as she did, she is hooked. It happens all the time.

Augie

PS. May the orphans of the world find their mother imagos. In this sense, as I explained to Barb, we are all orphans.

One more aside: Barb and I were talking about family origins. Shortly before, I had mentioned I was Jewish. She asked me where my grandparents were from. I stumbled and fumbled. Good analyst that she now is, she asked, "Are you embarrassed about their origins? I know they were Jewish." I have more work to do on my analysis than she does on hers.

Dear B. J.,

I have seen Barb once since the encounter. She is continuing with her rumination and is virtually on her own with analysis. Since our last meeting, she has been getting ready to leave for Seattle to see her mother. Since childhood, Barb has kept elaborate scrapbooks of her life. These last weeks, she has been feverishly getting them into shape. When I asked her why she was doing this, she said, "You know and I know—for my mother."

In our conversation, she asked me whether or not her car's breaking down this week was caused by her inclination not to go to see her "real" mother. "How can the mechanical breakdown of a car be related?" She asked the question feeling that she was in some way responsible. At this point in our conversations, I preferred not to make the analysis with her; but in the Hassidic mode, I illustrated with a story how the process might work.

One of the methods most effective in getting to my it is the reading of stories by those like Groddeck or Freud who do analyses. In reading them, my mind begins to wander and associations begin to fly. Just as my story might help Barb analyze why her car broke down, so her mention of her car's breaking down made me think anew about an incident that had happened to me. This incident, let us call it the "jockstrap incident," I will relate to you. I told it to Barb to help her with her analysis, and in the process, I learned a great deal more about my own incident. No doubt as I reopen the incident in this letter, I will learn even more. What I tell you here is more than I related to Barb. The point of the story is to show how we may be responsible for events that seem to be in the hands of another person, in the control of another force, or even in the mechanism of a machine.

My mother's birthday was coming up soon. Usually my wife and I together pick out a gift for my mother. I may pick out other people's presents, but I no longer look at it as accidental that selecting my mother's present gives me difficulty. This year I decided to select her gift by myself. I looked through the many catalogs we get and decided to pick out a terrycloth robe for her. The nicest one was in the Moss Brown runner's catalog. The thought occurred to me that I had better be right in my choice for there was little else in the catalog she might order if the robe did not suit her. I called up to order the robe and decided to place an order for myself as well. What was unusual was that the man taking the order was not too bright. Usually the people who take orders are alert, professional, and helpful. I ordered my running gear in preparation for winter: a pair of runner's briefs with a polypropylene front that looks like rubber to protect against cold, a face mask, and runner's tights. I carefully repeated the order and my address. I was aware of how careful I was in placing the order for I felt the clerk could botch it easily. When I placed the order for the robe, I gave my mother's address. The order clerk said they were out of stock. I told him to forget the order for the robe and just send the running gear to me. I ordered the robe for my mother a few days later from another catalog. I told my wife how inefficient the order clerk had been and emphasized how careful I had been in giving the order. I also expressed hope that he would get it right.

You can guess the rest. On a Saturday morning, the phone rang and my wife picked it up. The caller was my mother. Carole said, "I think you had better speak to Augie." My mother told me she had received this strange gift from me. She opened up the package and saw this huge pair of briefs, too big for her, with a rubber front. She wondered if I had sent them to her because I thought she was incontinent. At her age, many people have bladder problems. Then she saw the face mask and thought she could wear it to cover any shame she might feel from wearing the pants. Needless to say we were all hysterical. I have not laughed like that in years.

When we got off the phone, I asked Carole if my mother had seemed angry. Carole said that she gave me the phone because there was a cold tone on the other end of the line. My mother told me on the phone, "We are even now." Several years ago she sent me a birthday card in haste. It said, "To a Good Friend." We had gotten a hearty laugh from that.

The incident of the running gear was on my mind for the rest of the day. I told the story to several people and at other times broke out laughing from just thinking about it. As it was, I thought of it as a funny story only. Carole, weary of being reminded by me how we are responsible for our illness and actions, insisted I must have done it on purpose. She had turned my mother's call over to me knowing that I had goofed. I denied my complicity for a while, repeating how meticulous my instructions had been to the order clerk. I made no errors to him; I repeated everything at least twice. The tables were turned on me for I was protesting my innocence.

In private, I began to rethink the whole incident. (Tough to do in the presence of an "I told you so" analyst.) This was not the first time this type of incident had happened. Years ago when my wife and I were dating, I suggested that we buy our mothers cloth coasters that fit on the bottoms and up the sides of glasses. They were little jockstraps. Carole agreed. My mother was upset by the present. Carole had bought her mother flowers as well. She swears that she told me she was going to buy flowers, but I have always denied it, blaming Carole for the PR snafu. Now I can remember her telling me.

I began to think about my Moss Brown order. The clerk was obviously incompetent. I even thought of withdrawing my order so no mistake would be made. Why had I not called in each order separately to avoid confusion? Moss Brown has a toll-free number. These and similar thoughts were going through my mind as I ordered. My conclusion now is that despite the accident many years ago and the possibilities for a current mixup, I wanted a mixup to occur. The clerk had to perform his part, and I knew there was the chance that he would goof up. I set him up to be the villain in this piece. He came through. If he had not, I would have found another way to get back at my mother.

I did not have to look far for a motive. A week before I called in the order, my parents had called and told me about their visit with my sister in England. My "poor" sister and her husband had bought a new house. They were in the process of tearing the insides out and rebuilding it. As you know, "poor" images of my sister do not sit well with me, so I placed my order with Moss Brown using the order as a possible revenge and hiding behind the clerk's incompetence.

When I finished telling Barb my story, lights had already lit up. She had known for a long time that her car was not working properly. These last few weeks she had thought about the car quite often. Like my clerk, the car obliged and now the accelerator would not work properly. Besides, the tires are in poor condition and should be replaced before a long trip. Now she will have to delay the trip to find her "real" mother.

I fear for her safety and need to tell her so. Barb's story reminds me of a friend who made a decision to return to school. The decision was difficult because it involved running away from family, friends, and community. She was "hurrying" to get last minute chores done and ran through an intersection. The pickup she was driving was totaled. Luckily, she was not hurt and her father insisted on driving her to the university. Barb and I connived with our environment and brought the desired results: a delay in Barb's trip and an insult to my mother. (Fortunately for my other friend, she did not succeed in her purpose; she did not stay home. Perhaps she did get her way, however; her father drove her to school.)

I must tell you that I am withholding something from my story. As you probably guessed, there is more to the "jockstrap incident," my "poor" sister, and my mother's reaction. More details would be too embarrassing for the other parties involved. Since you know them both, I will refrain from giving the information. This does not take away from my story, however. If we teeter on the last rung of a ladder, speed through a yellow light, or balance six bags of groceries in our arms, we are, as the saying goes, "asking for it."

Please take care and beware of making anyone or anything an accomplice in your actions.

Angie

Dear B. J.,

It is interesting that you, too, are narrowing down the realm of chance. Let me repeat your example of the spaghetti dinner and see what else it suggests. You were having an old boyfriend over for dinner and were preparing your favorite recipe. You were pregnant—interesting you should mention it—and carried the bowl of spaghetti which was neither heavy nor full. You dropped it. Now you realize that there seemed to be no reason to drop it. Afterwards you spent hours cleaning it up, and you cooked another batch to show you could do it. Now you recognize how clever our it can be. I watch for facial expressions of those who tell me about an accident or illness. They become children all over again with sheepish or malicious expressions on their faces. So I imagine you reacting in these ways when you recalled your story.

If you want to go further in analyzing the incident, dwell on the consequences you mention: the cleanup and repeating the dinner. Let other consequences float into your mind. Curious also that you reveal your pregnancy. I must restrain myself from guessing and ask you to think about the circumstances some more.

I will leave you to those thoughts and switch to another subject you inquired about. I do need to elaborate on problems of writing and communication. They have been neglected in my formal writings, and my only mention of them to you was about the curse. I do need to expound on them for you are correct; they are important to my ideas. A number of years ago, I wrote a paper called "Why I Hate to Write." Only a few years ago, I gave a talk on the subject. Until I lifted the curse, writing was an obsession with me. I am not sure I have answered all my questions, but here are my tentative conclusions.

Writing is merely one form of communication to others. All our gestures, tics, illnesses, and injuries are also communications.

These are all presentations to others regardless of whether those people are present or not. I have spent a great deal of time testing this idea with myself and with others. In my letters to you, I come up with instance after instance where we look at the consequence of some activity and find it is a presentation to others. You can see this yet again in my suspicion that the "great spaghetti disaster" was aimed at some audience.

You may point to certain exceptions and say that sharpening a pencil or washing dishes is not a communication. My answer would be that when you were sharpening the pencil, you were doing so to make it easier to write something to someone. I may wash dishes to seek someone's praise, communicate to someone that I do my share of the dishes, or wash them to avoid chastisement. A Jamesian response to these instances might be that I no longer think about these activities and they are merely reflex. Yet, habits are built on purposes, and because we no longer remind ourselves each time we do something why we do it does not mean that purpose is no longer in our actions.

The person for whom we perform an act does not have to be present when we are performing it. Perhaps we think the person will find out from someone else about the activity we perform. Or that person may walk in the house and see the dishes have been washed. These seem to be obvious possibilities. But what if we are communicating with a parent or relative who does not even live in the state? We retain the possibility of telling them at some future date that we do the dishes, help around the house.

Communication can be direct as when we speak to the person in the room. I would even call it direct if we sprain an ankle in a person's presence and engage his or her sympathy. We also communicate indirectly in two ways. One is where our communication—the dishes or a letter—is left where the other person is bound to see it. Sometimes we are straightforward and post a letter; at other times we may leave it lying about. A friend of mine has a rule of thumb which I half admire, half abhor. If the children are obvious in leaving their letters and diaries around, she will read them. Her assumption is that one takes care to put what is confidential in a drawer. If a letter is left about, the child's intention is for an adult to read it. I was never willing to accept this, but in light of my own theories, she is probably right. We can write a diary to ourselves, but if it is out in the open, we want it to be read by other occupants of the house.

We communicate directly when we make certain another person is receiving the message. At other times, we communicate indirectly by leaving the message lying about. The second way we communicate indirectly is by reserving the right to report on an activity at some future time. In this sense, our actions which we can report to others are history. "Last week I hurt my foot playing ball." "I did the dishes twice last week." You are right, B. J., that I may be stretching my assumption. You could challenge me and say that only in conversations with others do I "recall" what happened and decide to communicate it to others. I suggest that much as Augie March in Saul Bellow's book is conscious of writing his own history (presumably for others), we engage in acts that are potential communications, and our it thinks of them as such. This is why they are so easily recollected.

In my language, direct means dropping a message in someone's lap, and indirect means leaving it lying about to be found or holding it in reserve for a later time. There is another dimension we might want to think about: are we aware of making the communication or is the communication in the province of the it? When you dropped the spaghetti, your message might have been directed at someone in the room, but you obviously were not aware of the communiqué. In Groddeck's language, your it was speaking to the other person's it. Much of my work, of course, is to expand our awareness on such matters in order to know ourselves better. For instance, I can always tell my standing with a relative by the presents I receive. As I explained to my children, when one person is angry with me, she goes to the dumpster in back of a K-Mart to forage for a shirt to send me. By the way, thank you for the lovely apple you sent me. It was perfection! Now think of the implications. My imagination runs wild and I am flattered.

Communications do not have to be made to a "real" person. In one sense, we may see the person and communicate directly to him or her, or communicate to an unknowable God, imaginary friend, or a cricket sitting on our shoulder. Many writers, including Gabriel Marcel, tell of having imaginary companions as a child. In all these cases, from the real to the imaginary, the recipients are our creations. Whether they are directly in front of us or in a storybook, we imagine how they will respond to us, how they will process the information, and how they will see us. All people, factual or fictional, are at least partially our creations. Perhaps all of those we meet are created by us in the image of our childhood companions, presumably mother and father, and possibly siblings. The more abstract the person, the more unknown to us, the more we can build into these primary relations. God is the father, sometimes the mother. All communications may be reductive and simply conversations with our parents. Even if we believe in such reductivism, we are still creating those we communicate with, whether Barb is creating her adoptive mother or I am creating a mother imago to speak with.

At times I am convinced by the reductive argument. People we meet and create are simply variants of those we knew or imagined when we were very young. I am not willing to go out on a limb for this view. It has been my practice, however, whether in dreams, in search of the cause of illness, or in everyday conversation, to check on the possibilities that the one I am speaking to is a stand-in or symbol for someone else. More importantly, they are our fictions, more or less, and we imagine much of the conversation that might follow. The key here is the ability to believe in the characters we create. In self-analysis, I can conjure up people and have them answer questions. This is no more than the strategy we try when we devise a plan for dealing with other people. They are, at least partially, our creations. I do not mean to sound dogmatic in this letter. Much as I take as a working hypothesis the idea that the it is the source of illness, so I take the idea that all our actions are communications to others. All of these others are creations of our own in some ways.

I will end this letter here, but leave you with some thoughts about my next letter. Surely between now and then you will be looking for some counterinstances. You will realize that I have not addressed whether there is "pure thought," what a conversation with oneself entails, or how all of this fully bears on written communication. Until next time I will be thinking of you as I have described above.

Augie

PS. For you, as you are and as I see you.

Dear B. J.,

You anticipated the tough questions, and it is easy for you
to see now why I put them off. Are we always social beings?
Do our actions at all times represent a communication to others?
Hannah Arendt in her last books on thinking and willing attempts
to speak of pure thought. Time and hence life can be sus-
pended. In my own meditations and those I read of others, there
appear to be no social objects. Yet, upon reflection, all my
thoughts seem to have social objects. Although as I write to you,
especially in these more analytical letters, I do lose sight of the
fact that I am writing to anyone at all. I am sure that when you
read my letters, or are writing your own, you "lose" yourself
and forget the object of the communication. "Pure thought" may
be when we suspend awareness through meditation or other activity and allow our it to express itself in fragments and wild
associations—much in the way I have been describing it-talk in
our letters. Our awareness captures many of these expressions
of the it as they cross our minds. At bottom, however, is a
rumination about another person, a social concern, or a communication to a living, dead, or imagined being, near or far. To
use a term of Gamaliel Bradford, we have pre-thinking here. A
rehearsal is on for future social activity. Meditation, free association, it-talk—whatever the concept you use—brings forth pre-
thinking which is concerned with how we address others.

Another instance of "losing" ourselves occurs when we are
engaged in an activity, like carpentry, at which we may be good
and are achieving excellence. Like Plato, let me speak here of
the simpler trades. When I work on building a cabin, I can work
for hours and not realize how much time has passed. I am con-
centrating on the task at hand and "losing" myself in that task.
Is every nail I drive and every two by four cut a social act? There
is something rhythmical and habitual about these actions. The
easy answer is to say that every nail driven is the sex act, and

every cut an execution. In many ways this answer is true; thoughts like these are thoughts of the it. They pop into awareness every so often. But other thoughts intrude: how much more quickly I need to work to keep up with my partner; how pleased my wife will be to see my progress; what will we decide to do next. Every nail and every two by four remind me of something else. Every act is an action towards someone else, every act reminds me of the consequences of the act. To be "lost" in such an activity is to give free play to the it.

I do not want to cut off my finger or hammer my thumb, so free association is hindered by attentiveness to my job. Every nail is a threat to my fingers; the saw is a menace as well. I do not want to bring these injuries back to others. As I give you it-talk on carpentry, what becomes apparent is how active and social are those things we do. No, I cannot tell you what every knock with the hammer means, but even the most rhythmical jobs, ones which we "lose" ourselves in, are social. The act itself may be an expression of sexuality or aggression—and also reminds us of other consequences of our acts. Pretty radical I know, but stay with me for a while.

My friend Mike argues that we are always carrying on a dialogue with ourselves. In my terms, this can go on between life (the it) and awareness(the I), or in awareness as it is fed by contradictory streams of life. I only add that this inner dialogue is always with the other in mind.

Another circumstance I use to illustrate human sociability is the lonely trek an individual chooses to take up a dangerous peak. I pick this as an example, because I have always been fascinated by the loner "pitting himself or herself against nature." Also, I use this as an example because it seems as far away from a communication as any activity I could think of. When I have spoken at length with such a daredevil, I learn there is always a person at home for whom he is performing: a wife or mother, afraid for his life. What an attention grabbing device: go off on a dangerous mission! Recently, an acquaintance planned to go to the Himalayas and climb a peak from a side not yet conquered. Relatives read about the adventure in the papers and with concern called him on the phone. George Simmel, the philosopher-sociologist, suggests the ubiquity of social relations in his writings when he describes the status the stranger has within a group. The stranger is thought of even as the group forms and is an integral part of the group although not a member. The mountain climber is far from civilization, free, yet his or her actions are tied to those at home. He or she is aware of what others may be thinking and is busy manufacturing the dialogue to be used on return. Those climbers I have talked to at length get the sympathy and attention of people because others fear for the climbers' safety. Most dangerous to the climbers, of course, is their need to get hurt to engage someone's attention.

Emerson suggested that all nature is symbol for us. Climbing the mountain, reclining near the stream, looking up at the clouds—we see nature as we see others. In this sense as well, solitude may be a communication.

I am not sure that I convince you. But even if you show me pure thought, remember, as Rousseau reminded us, it was learned through others; language is a social convenience. We are reminded of others as we utter anything. As much as we try to dissolve ourselves in pure thought or pure being, we are communicating with others.

Now we are getting at some core ideas. I view the study of philosophy as an activity to advance the awareness of our possibilities, hence our freedom. At every stage of this activity, our autonomy is enhanced, even while we are reminded of limits to our freedom. For instance, Socrates instructs us that we, not the gods, must be sovereign in matters of discerning the truth. We take a great step towards autonomy, and yet Socrates' quest reminds us of the limits of freedom, the boundary conditions. In his quest to understand the Oracle of Delphi, he goes to show that we are ignorant and it is worse to presume we are knowledgable. Another boundary made clear for Socrates by his awareness is that once he is knowledgable, he must withdraw from politics. He must avoid the political arena because his autonomy would clash with the state. Socrates' contribution was to show the frontiers of freedom and hence how they point out how society may limit the individual in his or her pursuit of awareness.

Hence we have the dialectic of acknowledging our freedom with increasing awareness of our limits. I have no need to trace this history down to today. There is no surprise in the existentialists' tendency to stress choice and authenticity and to become acutely aware of its relationship with the boundary conditions of death. I am sure you know where I am leading. Freud and Groddeck, respectively, give us the unconscious and the it undermining our freedom. At the same time, knowledge of these conditions strengthens the I, enhances our freedom to act. In my own thought, isolation, quietude, a dialogue concerning only oneself, a solitary communion with nature all disappear. We are constantly expressing ourselves to others. Consequently, health now is in the realm of choice.

One way out of this is to prove me wrong, to prove that all our thoughts are not social and thus we are freer than I could even imagine. My position is that in the sense I talk about, we are social animals. Others are never far from our thoughts or actions. This is my working hypothesis. Perhaps I am saying that if you complete a thought or an action and say it is autonomous you simply have not looked deeply enough into the matter. Similarly, Freud argued with his detractors that when they found death in a dream, they had not looked far enough. Beneath this thought of death is a neurotic relationship with another. This is as far as I can carry my working hypothesis.

The prospects of partially losing my freedom, as this idea suggests, are not grave. As the unconscious, or the it, allowed Freud and Groddeck more control over their existence, so increasing awareness is liberating for me. What I want to know is to whom I am speaking. Once I realize every thought or action is a communication, I want to express myself with clarity and candor. The tragedies in the lives of Nietzsche and Sartre were the illusions of freedom they had. The big lie was that they kept themselves from seeing that the *ubermensch*, or the authentic choosing individual, was trying to express his freedom to others. "I am free" is the statement not to oneself but to others. Nietzsche ended his days as a complete burden to others and Sartre died of a stroke, the complete destruction of autonomy and reason. Perhaps I cannot accurately guess for others, but I am so intrigued by the possibilities I think someday I will do a Groddeckian analysis of their lives. Anyway, they enhanced our ideas of freedom and drew to our attention the boundaries of death. For me, all is communication with others, a condition that both takes away and enhances our freedom.

Augie

Dear B. J.,

Thanks for your comments on my last letter. You correctly point out one of my major differences with Groddeck. He tends to emphasize only the sides of his discoveries that take away from our freedom: we are fully governed by the it, consciousness is a trick of the it, etc. In my darker moments, I tend to agree with him, and the possibility remains for me that awareness is completely part of the it's chicanery. My approach, however, is to begin with the concept of awareness and try to wrest as much from life as I can. This may ultimately be a losing process, but I prefer to struggle towards awareness. Groddeck tends to emphasize just the opposite. He ignores or minimizes his role in cure and ignores or minimizes especially the role of awareness. His writings, particularly *The Book of the It,* are often written to appeal to the it of another. Yet there is the Groddeck who writes books, appeals to awareness, and desires recognition from at least Freud and maybe others.

One of the dimensions of character, from my book of the same name, is a *return* which means that a person with character returns to the world on his or her own terms. How does this reconcile with the idea that all our actions are communications to others? To further the notion of return, one must return knowing that all is a communication and whom one is addressing, what we wish to tell that person, and to whom one wishes to speak next. I explained to you my assumption that all is communication, and perhaps I can now illustrate the process by example. My correspondence illustrates how all is communication, both by addressing you as an individual as well as by showing how illness and other behavior is communication.

I choose to speak here of writing as communication, not of carpentry or other skills. Even though writing as communication seems to be a cliché, we never make this process as clear as we could. A student of mine asked me to critique her writing.

She told me that her style seemed verbose and she took too long getting to the point. She is a social worker and is not very efficient in turning in reports on clients. Her written work for my class seemed to prove her point because it included everything I would want to know, she would want to know, or any reasonable person would ever want to know. We got around to the consequences of her writing, and she said it was to please me as well as herself. When discussion moved to the social work reports she does, it turns out that she is writing to several parties. She is writing to her supervisor who wants certain standard information that can be compared with what is in the reports of others. At the same time, she is writing to the lawyer who may question in court someday her judgment of the client. This may have no useful purpose within the agency. Finally, she is writing for herself. Her own writing will help her in her daily dealings with the client. In my language, these notes are for her client, not for her, and are part of an ongoing dialogue with the client.

When she saw the many audiences she was addressing, it became obvious to her why her case notes were so difficult to compose. Knowing this, she may be able to cut down on her notes. More importantly, she will know whom she is addressing and, therefore, her writing will become more direct and incisive. You can see my general inclinations, and as you might expect, if I were doing this analysis on myself, I would see if those I assumed I was writing for were possible stand-ins for someone else.

Only recently have I understood the full implications of these ideas. In *Character,* I began to look back at earlier writings as a record of my unconscious thoughts. Now I look to see whom I was addressing. No wonder writing is so difficult. On superficial glance, even then, I thought I was writing for a large audience and applause; a committee of peers who might judge me for tenure; in a general way, friends and relatives; and finally, myself, whatever that meant. As I look back and analyze the situation, my audience was my wife/mother and father. As I explained earlier, my father had cursed me. I could never write. Those who would read and review my works were males who would look down with skepticism on my work and abilities. My father figuratively occupied a desk in the publisher's office and sat on the tenure and promotion committees. Many writers harbor secret thoughts of "popularity," mass appeal. Today this may be expressed as hoping to appear on TV: twenty years ago it was an appearance on the "Tonight Show," now it is an appearance on "Good Morning, America."

These delusions of grandeur I had thought for a long time were merely cultural; in democracies, as described by de Tocqueville, truth is acceptance by the masses. When I saw these delusions in others, I was willing to accept them as the cultural norm. Upon further scrutiny, I found that we speak to one person at a time. If we engage a crowd, we do so with one person in mind. Although many people may read my writings, I often select my mother as my "audience." However, my mother never reads my work. Of course, if I wrote a "best seller," others would induce her to do so. Contrast her behavior toward my writing with her behavior toward my successful amateur basketball career. My mother was intensely interested in my athletic achievements; therefore, because I played to her and she responded, I was indifferent to the acclaim or size of the rest of the audience. Since I held her interest, I needed no crowd to convey anything to her.

At this time, I am not willing to say that mass appeal means the same to everyone. My suspicion is, after talking with many, that each of us speaks to one person in a crowd, exhorts the crowd in order to reach that "important" one, or fears the crowd will convey a negative impression to the "important" one.

As I look over my writings, I can see that the same piece may address several different individuals. In *Character* I was developing the idea of *mensch,* a concept that my father taught me obliquely, and I was hoping it would please him. At other times, I was scolding him for lacking in certain virtues. Friends were the models for the enthusiast, the ironic person, and other characters I drew. I was telling them what they were and how they might change. My mother was the model for other types of character in the book; I was hoping she would read the volume. Many others trotted into those pages, objects of my descriptions, so that I could teach them better ways or warn others about them.

Let me make a few points before I mislead you completely. My book does not reduce or dissolve to a purely personal statement. I do not recant what I said in *Character* about the public situation and the "flawed" characters that constitute the situation. I still see them out there, but this public situation was rendered from portraits of those I know and directly communicate with. Perhaps I even rendered some by carrying on imaginary conversations with public figures and those others known only through my reading. I may be scolding the criminal I do not know. Most likely, however, he or she resembles one close by. I understood some of this at the time of my writing for I spoke of valuative empiricism, which means that knowledge of the public situation is governed by knowledge of yourself and the public situation.

When I wrote *Character* and other works, I was not as conscious of my audiences as I am now. When I was writing in the past, it was far more difficult. I was cursed, and those who I felt would read my work were skeptical judges. In paranoid terms, I did not know my accusers. Until I identified my audience, writing was far more difficult. In the example of the student which I gave earlier, she did not know, was not aware of, her audience. Once you are aware, you may confront, exhort, criticize that person or persons directly. If that person is difficult to address, you now ask the questions: Why? How can I best convey what I want? Should I ignore that person and not answer, or should I boldly convey my ideas to him or her? Facing an audience unknown to awareness is like Kafka's K facing his unknown accusers. In *The Writer and Psychoanalysis,* Edmund Begler speaks of writing as a justification. In my terms, it is a way to give sympathy or slay one's antagonists. This is far more difficult to do when you do not know who they are.

Yes, my letters are addressed to you and you are my audience. What is true, however, is that as I cover different topics, my audience can change. The last letter I wrote was very difficult for in it was a confrontation with Groddeck as well as writing to you, a friend. Yes, the letter was to you, but the difficulty came in addressing Groddeck as well. As you know, there was a gap between the last letter and the one before. Knowing before I started the letter that I was confronting him would have made my writing easier.

In talks and essays before reading Groddeck, I had always contrasted difficulties in writing with difficulties in speech. Speech was always easier for me, and I felt this was because I was confronted in writing by my own words. Verbal messages, in contrast, vanished into thin air. Now I see that speech can be difficult as well. You may be speaking to a friend, but getting in a dig at a relative. An oral presentation to a large audience may be carried to the ears of others not in the audience. Speech, however, does have the advantage of directness. There is an audience before you. Even if the talk is formulated for someone else as well, you are directing it to a person or persons. Effective public speakers before a large audience will invariably talk to a person, real or imagined, not to all of the audience.

Writing, as Simmel suggests, means that a secret is out and is available to others. It can potentially be read by someone a continent away. Before I was aware of these principles, I began to fill notebooks, for myself, of my thoughts. They were social for they were all directed at someone, but by keeping them for myself they were only potential messages to others, therefore not as threatening to me. Writing for yourself is not truly for yourself, but potentially for others.

I have not talked about why we may have intense feelings about how our writing is received and perhaps lesser feelings about our carpentry or reading or skiing. You have to remember that you and I, unlike most in society, make our living through our writing. Writing is our virtue, and persons from our present as well as our future will judge us on our writing. If they judge me on my skiing, less is at stake, for I am not prone to concern myself with such judgments. I am more sensitive about whether I am or am not a good writer. More of myself is wrapped up in such judgments. My policemen students are uninhibited writers. Their careers depend on judgment and action, and they could care less about how their writing is evaluated.

In many ways, those brought up in the culture, policemen excepted, find writing difficult even if it is not their occupation. Part of this is living as Kafka's K and delivering messages to the unknown. Moreover, we are nurtured/murdered in public schools that constantly judge us on our writing skill. Let me give you an example which occurred with our son Martin, which illustrates some of these points. Before bed the other night, he gave me a short story he had written for class. I seem to be his censor in much the way my father was for me. He always gives me his papers to read when I am in a hurry or about to fall asleep. If I were to guess for him, I would say that he chooses such times because he can then discount my judgment as hurried or distorted by torpor. You know I try to be nonjudgmental, but he demands to know his worth as a writer. When I make my corrections and impress upon him that I am correcting to the truth in some platonic way and not judging his ultimate worth as a writer, he still takes my comments as judgmental.

The next morning he brought the paper to Carole, another important audience, and asked her to read it. The only problem was that she had to leave for work in five minutes and refused to read it. Two minutes later she went to brush her teeth and found the bathroom locked and our son holding siege. Rarely does he use this particular bathroom. He wanted his mother to read the paper, in haste of course, and she refused. She got upset over his monopoly of the bathroom. He roundly accused her of losing her temper and wagging an uncivil tongue. In effect, he was criticizing her for not reading his paper. He wanted our response. As well, writing was an important judgment on his worth. He was using his short story as a barometer of his future success in the film industry. As I did so many times in the past, he made the double error of not directly knowing whom he was addressing in the paper, nor did he refrain from judging himself through the eyes of the other.

No, I am not angry with him, nor is Carole. Before reflection, it passes as a minor incident to all. Yet this made up part of Martin's rumination for the day if not the year. Such are the ways of life, of the it. Bringing this to his awareness, or better still, allowing him to reflect on these events in his own way, we try to help him become captain of his consciousness. I begin with this possibility. Groddeck seems to act on this assumption, but will not acknowledge it.

Augie

PS. As you can see by this last sentence, the letter was directed to you and Georg Groddeck, as well as others I could identify. Say hi to my mom and tell her how clever I am.

Dear B. J.,

I believe you are sincere when you say that you write for yourself. Let me make a few comments on this state of affairs before I tantalize you with some other ideas. If I take it on face value that you write for yourself, you do not contradict my ideas about communication. You describe this self of yours as accepting, yet critical in a positive way. This "you" is a self imago, a fiction you have created out of all your possibilities. This imago is no different in structure from the God you perform for, the mother imago, the cricket on your shoulder, or a character in a book. I have known past B. J.'s who were sarcastic and hypercritical or, on the other hand, warm, generous, and overly accepting. (The present B. J. has certainly shown the latter characteristics with respect to my ideas.) So you see, your self imago is a fictional person you are talking to. I would suggest that you probe deep down to see if this self imago is not someone else disguised as your image. Use it-talk as you think about your imago. I am sure that the imago, as you state it, will be someone else, an imago that will please someone else, or as George Herbert Mead might have it, an amalgam of the hoped for expectations of others.

All through my letters I have used the word *sympathy* and hinted that the consequence of illness is gaining the sympathy of others. Here I must indicate my departure from Groddeck. In all of his works, he asks people to look at the consequences of their illnesses. Illnesses are metaphors the it creates to communicate. This it of Groddeck's is sometimes straightforward and helpful; people avoid activities they do not want to participate in by getting sick. At other times the it is devilish or, in Groddeck's terms, like a troll, making mischief. He talks of the woman who upon seeing asparagus in a basket, falls down and breaks her leg. He writes his letters as Patrik Troll and tends to side with the view of the it as a troll. Constantly, however, these images shift from helpful to malevolent to mischievous.

In an article called "The It and Disease," Groddeck tries to catalog many of the ways in which the it creates symptoms. The function of a symptom is to produce certain consequences. He always speaks of consequences of symptoms in the plural, not the singular. I can discern several consequences, described in this article, of the its creation of illness. To be sick is to be a child again and all powerful. The child who is sick gains much attention. All sorts of people minister to the ill. Granted, B. J., this is not the power to direct others' every action towards a given goal, but it is the power to command the attention of others and direct them to help you.

A related point for Groddeck is that life for the child begins with the mother, and after separation from the mother, the child is forever trying to return to her. To be ill and a child is to summon the mother. In most of Groddeck's writings, people are responding to and returning to the mother. The power of illness is to induce others to help, others who are in some sense the mother. B. J., my analyses of myself and others tend to confirm this idea, but in my writings I wish to pose no such definite structure. Otherwise my students, in their enthusiasm to agree with me, would find *my* structures, not their own.

Groddeck suggests other consequences of illness. The person who is sick has no consciousness of guilt, or at least the illness may temporarily destroy guilt. All the sick person can think about is his or her misery. This brings about yet another point by Groddeck. The illness is a punishment in itself, a way of expiating sin. A sickness is a way to make the universe compensatory, a mechanism that Emerson so well described. A person gets ill and feels he is even. He has harmed another and the universe has gotten even with him. Finally, an illness is a means of repression. An individual postpones dealing with a conflict or drives it so deep into the it that she does not have to deal with it again.

Throughout his writings, Groddeck sprinkles suggestions about the "personality of the it" and the consequences of illness. When I ask myself the consequences of my own illnesses, I free myself for it-talk. I may let my mind wander over the possibilities that Groddeck suggests. Rarely, however, do I get anywhere by going over, in cookbook fashion, the possible answer. Groddeck, in his article "The It and Disease," was summarizing findings, not teaching method. What I do ask myself, and it is effective, is, What are the consequences of my illness? I interpret this to mean that the illness is a communication to another; I am asking for sympathy. Who comes to mind that I would like to tell of my illness? What would I tell that person? What would his or her reaction be? If the it-talk about consequences does not yield answers, answers to these general probes usually do.

Let me explain my methods and my differences with Groddeck. He assumes illness is a symbol and has a cause interna. The consequences of illness, as described above, are many and varied. When he theorizes about the process, he remains open, if not reverent, and even mystical. Perhaps this is the best that can be done on the matter. What I suggest is that we are looking for sympathy and communicating this to another. In my theory, all of the consequences are distilled as pleas for sympathy. Of course, the person we are speaking to need not be present; the disease may be an indirect summons to another.

B. J., I think if you will look at Groddeck with me you will find that his explanations are not inconsistent with my views about sympathy. The sick child is going to draw others to him or her through sympathy and concern. By sympathy I mean a feeling of oneness with another, a concert of concern, an identity. Watch children and you will see how, through illness, they draw the attentions of others like a magnet. More interesting, watch the faces of the concerned sympathizers. You can then see what it means to win from losing, or getting sympathy when ill. Needless to say, in most families, the mother will come running when the child is sick. When my children were growing up, I understood this dynamic. I tried to give them as little sympathy as I could. The child is crafty; and in such situations, he or she can escalate illness, make you feel bad, or point out your "psychopathic" behavior to a third party to get that party to make you volunteer sympathy. I have explained the child in us to others, and they say, "You are wrong, all I want is to be left alone when ill." Invariably I ask them if anyone else knows they are ill; do they have someone they would like to inform; do they enjoy others sympathizing with their illness and admiring how brave they are to face the illness alone? This last ploy was *my* personal strategy. I would suffer in silence to an unseen audience who would applaud my stoic courage.

Groddeck's other findings are not inconsistent with my views. For instance, you may be asking for sympathy from your mother. Also, not only does illness erase in your own mind the guilt for a wrong deed, but it also allows sympathy to override the anger others feel toward you because of your wrong deed. How many times have you heard people say something like, "I don't like X, but you have to feel sorry for him (her). What a terrible illness." Illness is a punishment you inflict on yourself to expiate guilt. If Groddeck is correct, you can see why it is so difficult to give up explaining illness by external cause. If you give up this explanation, then you remain guilty and unworthy of sympathy.

Finally, for Groddeck, an illness is a means of delaying thoughts about guilt or driving it deep into the it. Through repression you try to convince yourself that you still have the sympathy of others.

What I suggest then is that all illnesses are communications of sympathy to others, a part of the more general notion that all behavior is a communication to others. These communications are to ask people for sympathy. When I found myself challenging that idea, I found myself very angry with another person and getting sick over the incident. Upon reflection, and I will tell you more of this next time, I appeared to have two choices: regaining the *sympathy* of or *annihilating* that person. One of the ways to sympathy is to make the other person sorry that you are ill (translation of it to it: "You should be sorry for making me ill and should apologize") or to annihilate that person from your world and consciousness. The latter is more difficult and has severe costs.

Keep in mind that illness is only one strategy for capturing sympathy, the one I have dwelled on in these letters. I save these observations on communication, sympathy, and annihilation until after other considerations because, although they help to understand the dynamics of my philosophy, they become a bit technical. At this point I try to close the circle on my philosophy, working as Ortega did, on successive approximations to the truth. The tighter the approximations become, the more technical I become and I am afraid I might lose my reader. In my next letter, I will continue on this line of discussion, but try to lighten up a bit. My letters are beginning to resemble my lectures.

Augie

PS. Motto in doctor's office should be: Stay well. If you want my sympathy or anyone else's, please be direct and ask for it.

Dear B. J.,

Thanks for your encouragement. I will continue in my discussion of the terms *sympathy* and *annihilation*. When I speak of sympathy, I speak of the same phenomenon as does Martin Buber. Sympathy occurs when one is not categorizing or defining the other person or object. The individual is at one with the other. This sympathy can be looked at as the object of communication. Much of the time, as I have pointed out, this oneness may be brought about by the it. Through illness, we create a sympathetic bond with the other. (Sometimes sympathy drapes over into pity, a less desirable state.) We are, at least temporarily, at one with the other.

Another way we have of reacting is to try to annihilate the other person as a way of ridding ourselves of a state of tension. If the other disappears, then we do not remain in conflict. The goal, as Saint Augustine might say, is peace through war. If sympathy cannot be won through direct or indirect communication, accord can be reached by submission or disappearance of the other.

Most of the time, B. J., we live in limbo, neither in full sympathy nor with full power of annihilation. Walter Kaufmann disagrees with Buber and feels that we are often in concert with others. I tend to side with Buber for whom such sympathetic feelings are fleeting. We vacillate between feelings of sympathy and annihilation, but exist mostly in between, ill at ease with existence. In open and direct communication with others, we are aware of the condition that Camus called *little-ease*. We are not at one with others, past, present, or future, and we cannot do a permanent job of annihilation of others, either through outward force or inward repression. Concerning inward repression, Groddeck contented that we could drive our thoughts so deep into the recesses of the it that they might never surface again. I wish I could be so sure.

217

What we can hope for is to fully and openly express ourselves to others. The *differences* between ourselves and others must be manifest, appreciated, and respected. These differences and our appreciation of them are life, or little-ease, in between polarities of annihilation and sympathy which lie on the boundaries of our existence and represent death. Radical notions, I know, B. J.

Let me see if I can shed more light on these distinctions. Annihilation is not difficult to see as death. Life is the communication with all that is around us. At death we may sever our relationship with those who surround us. We can imagine our enemies dead, silent, or banished. In many cases our desire to annihilate others comes from fear that they might act upon us first. While jogging one day and being in a state of reverie, another jogger stepped in front of me as if I did not exist. Because he did not want to recognize my existence, my response was to render him nothing—and did so through murderous urges. When someone does not recognize our existence, we have two polar choices: winning the other to sympathy or annihilating him or her. Both can be difficult to live with: the former involves the scheming of the it to flatter, to plot, or as we have discussed so often, to become ill; the latter uses murderous fantasies.

We often try the option of annihilation but fall short. Annihilation is impractical and does not work unless we can satisfy ourself through dreams, vicarious revenge, or actual injury or annihilation of the other. Those whom we wish to annihilate can fight back tenaciously. In one of Saul Bellow's stories, he shows the power of a person who wishes to be recognized. He says that his character, an overweight woman, has been ignored by others, treated as if she does not exist. Her revenge is to be so loud, so demanding of people, that nobody can deny her existence. In total annihilation of others rests the hope for peace, but short of that goal, partial annihilation forces communication. Like Bellow's character, most people will resist annihilation. This resistance is communication and, therefore, life, as opposed to death.

The other direction in which we can move is towards sympathy. In my other letters, B. J., I tell of anger towards others or others' anger towards me; and if I am not careful, in order to effect reconciliation, I will move towards sympathy by seeking illness. With someone who is not in sympathy with me, I can choose to annihilate that person or bring him or her towards sympathy. I was speaking with a friend yesterday who in our conversation was reflecting both poles. He kept talking of leaving the town he has lived in for nineteen years. His children were growing up; perhaps he could get another job. Alternately, he spoke of challenges in town, his competitiveness, and his desire to succeed. As well, he spoke of liking the town, always getting along with the people, and making do for the rest of his life. I could not imagine what was at the bottom of this. Near the end of the conversation, it all came out. A person who had been his friend for nineteen years had disagreed with him recently, and yesterday my friend had underscored their personal differences in a heated argument. My friend said to me that the town was not big enough for the two of them. One would be driven out. Then he spoke of how reasonable they had been with one another in the past and how he hoped for reconciliation. He was pre-thinking strategies of annihilation and sympathy. I hope he does not choose to get ill in the near future.

So you see, we have the two alternatives: annihilation and sympathy. In the former alternative, we can suppress or eliminate what we do not like in the other person. Perhaps once the undesirable characteristics are nullified by fantasy, physical distance, violence, or restraint, our existence becomes easier. In the latter alternative, through illness or manipulation, we win the other person over to our side.

Why do I speak of both annihilation and sympathy as borders of death? We carry two contrasting images of death: one of annihilation and the other of sympathy. In the former image, we cease to exist. We are no more; we are nothingness. As Edgar Allan Poe describes in his essay on poetry, there is no darker word than *nevermore.* It is the cessation of a relationship with others and the world. In the latter image, we have sympathy, the destruction of difference between the self and others. We are the other person; we are the universe. This also is death. It is the cessation of difference; we are at one with another, our mother, the earth, the universe. The latter circles around the former, sympathy becomes annihilation, to be everything is to be nothing. More comforting views, as Miguel de Unamuno so acutely points out, involve a life after death, a continued differentiated existence. Hell for Unamuno is more comforting than death because, in my terms, it points to a relationship. Annihilation and complete sympathy involve a total destruction of relationship and dialogue.

What do we then strive for? In Eastern religions, it appears to be death, for if we can speak of goals in Zen and Hinduism (an obvious problem to use the term *goal* here), we speak of annihilation of feelings for the world as we know it and total sympathy with the universe. More and more as I think of the problems of existence, I see this as a possibility for all of us. We are striving through annihilation or sympathy for death. Most practitioners of the Eastern arts I know are existentialists who value their own individuality. So go the rhythms of philosophy. As we find our individuality, search for its possibilities, so its limits appear as death. The existentialists protest too much about death. They fear death because it is comfortable, a reconciliation with others, as well as terrible.

Why do I bring all this up? Because my hypothesis is that when we get sick we do it to ourselves. A moderate proposition is that death is a consequence of the it's not understanding that death may be a consequence of illness. Now you can anticipate my conclusion here. Sympathy is the wish for reconciliation, for death. Illness brings rest and is a metaphor for death. Beware also of the it handling death in still another way. Death is a way of settling our accounts, a way of drawing the ultimate in sympathy from another human being: a tear on our grave.

How then do we act? We move towards sympathy with others while recognizing differences. We can never be one with another short of death. This is an insight of Georg Simmel. We must not judge others on the basis of how closely they sympathize with us. We must look at others as incomplete beings struggling to place awareness above the it. Understanding others is even more difficult than understanding ourselves for we have only indirect access to their its. What we see in others as sympathy or indifference may be partial manifestations of ruminations that they have and are unaware of. As best we can, we communicate to their purposes and move towards sympathy.

At the same time, we must recognize and value difference, a manifestation of our freedom and of life.

Wow! I never meant to go on like this. Perhaps all of this expresses my feelings towards you. In all of my letters, I move towards concert and sympathy with you. At first, your comments and criticisms cut sharply until I recognized the principle of difference. Your own views, so unlike mine, are interesting, careful, and very different from my own. This should be a cause for celebration. This is life, whereas total sympathy is death. In all my writings, since they are my lifework, you find the contrary tendencies of annihilation of opposition and fostering total sympathy. These death impulses give vitality to my writing. In all, I must settle for life, the respectful communication of difference.

Augie

Dear B. J.,

You are correct in suggesting that the self, communication, annihilation, sympathy, and difference, as well as many other concepts I develop would be sufficient if our lives were controlled by awareness. These concepts give us a recognition of difference to aim for when we expand awareness. At times, as with sympathy and communication, these concepts may even suggest methods for expanding awareness. They are more than guides to understanding; they imply methods to aid in full understanding. At any rate, I include them late in our correspondence, for they might influence too much what you find. As with Freud and Groddeck, I too get tempted to understand the mechanisms of behavior and to posit my system. I hope that my system is spare and unobtrusive enough so that those who read me do not find themselves coerced to my views.

If reason were fully captain, awareness alone the secret to behavior, I would give you these structures and nothing else. With my assumption that we begin with our awareness to capture life, I accept these structures, constantly questioning them as I delve into the it. As Groddeck might say, these structures could be a trick of the it, a personal statement of structures and needs.

On another subject, you see a key difference between myself and Groddeck. You and I can both conclude that he was keenly aware of himself and others. One can love him even as he admits to being self-interested, sadistic, blunt, unsympathetic, and a host of other traits we viewed in the past as negative. Recognition of these traits in himself and others makes him a person one can find difference with and grow to love. He did not fully acknowledge, however, his need for communication with and the recognition of others. In this sense, as with Sartre and Nietzsche, he did not push far enough.

In my last letter to you, I admitted my wish to annihilate others, to manipulate to get their sympathy. Only by constant reminders to myself and through discipline do I treat others with a principle of difference. That is, I respect them for the independent ideas they develop from our communication. Still, I am always tempted to say I taught B. J., or she learned from me. The urge for authorship is great—we could call it the need to impress on others our own views, a position pushing to annihilation—and it is irrepressible. Maimonides knew this when he suggested that the most admirable act of charity, and most rare, is the giving of a gift anonymously. In other words, as Albert Camus suggests, we are all gangsters.

As you know, *Guns and Garlic* was my first book and one I am very fond of. Years after writing it, I found out why I wrote it. The myth of the gangster is that he is all powerful, wealthy, and unlike most in society lives in close-knit sympathy with a community of accomplices. Annihilation is his style, and he can have what he wants. The Manichaean world of the gangster, however, turns out to be an ideal, a goal, and not a reality. The power of the gangster is limited. He cannot act with impunity or he loses the respect of others of his kind and brings violence on his own head. More than likely, a gangster spends most of what he takes in and lives in fear, not sympathy or community, with his fellow workers. Even the gangster is limited. Camus may be correct. We are all gangsters at heart, restrained by the social system.

I admit that I am in actuality a gangster, that I help you to cure yourself not out of altruism but perhaps out of a sense of annihilation of you and your basic ideas and that only through discipline can I aspire to rejoice in our difference. I say this so as not to shoot myself in the foot with you. I do so to suggest that until we search ourselves, admit what we are, and accept all as human, we are bound to each other in miscommunication and lack of understanding. I know it is an Enlightenment goal, but I rest on the idea that increasing knowledge of life through awareness enhances the possibility that we can effectively communicate difference to one another.

You can probably sense that I am wrapping up some unfinished business in this letter. This can never be done neatly, and I am continuing with my research, moving from consideration of sympathy and towards annihilation. I will continue to correspond, but I use this letter to finish off some rough edges.

I have invited you to consider my views and Groddeck's views. At times I may sound shrill because discovery that we can expand control of our own lives to include control of illness is exciting. Along with this discovery of our freedom, I find that we are always ill, planning to get ill, and are overwhelmed. Bacteria or a virus seems much more straightforward to deal with. The only way to stay on top is to discipline ourselves to deal with this reality. Along with freedom come limits.

Out of all of this comes the most exciting possibility. With respect to curing illness, everything works. Norman Cousins shows this in *Anatomy of an Illness,* as do Barbara Brown and Hans Selye in their work. The gangster in me has to remind you, however, that even though "everything works," until you reconcile life and awareness as I suggest, cure may be temporary and illness may return.

Finally, you can see my petulance in my letters. I am better than the others. They are my cousins, my sister, the ones that get the credit while I am rotten. Is it possible that all my letters come from petulance? Does my curiosity about the causes of illness stem from my conviction that my siblings used sympathy to gain the attention of my parents? Illness was their way of gaining sympathy, and I caught on to their game and used it with more subtlety and effectiveness. When I found Groddeck, there was no shock in learning of his ideas. My early thoughts about my family led to the same conclusions as his. Groddeck was a great help and comfort: a help in that he had thought through some of these ideas for me and a comfort in that his writings demonstrate I do not think in isolation, without a sympathetic friend. The more I look, the more I see others confirm the observations of Groddeck and Sayres. We learn to use illness to gain sympathy with others.

My correspondence with you and the report of your experiences add further confirmation. When the gangster in me "takes cover" (although is never "rubbed out"), I am thrilled that although you do not use my thinking and Groddeck's as we would, you have found your own way through issues like freedom and limits, autonomy and communication, sympathy and annihilation, and life and awareness. In the future I expect to be enriched by your difference and play the role of listener, not gangster. This is the ultimate discipline, the very definition of a teacher.

Augie